AF587555

Fast Facts for Healthcare Professionals

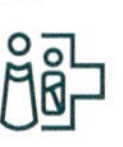

—

Women's and Children's Health

Early Hearing Detection and Intervention

EDITOR: Christine Yoshinaga-Itano[1]

Bianca Birdsey,[2] Emma Butcher,[3] Gwen Carr,[4] Shelly Chadha,[5] Hsiu-wen Chang,[6] Adrian C Davis,[7] Harald A Euler,[8] Elaine Gale,[9] Daniel Holzinger,[10] Cynthia Hunnicutt,[1] Lisa L Hunter,[11] Rachel Knowles,[3] Doris R Lewis,[12] Vinaya Manchaiah,[1] Philipp Mathmann,[8] Katrin Neumann,[8] Waheeda Pagarkar,[13] Allison L Sedey,[1] Tony KS Sirimanna,[13] Trudy Smith,[14] Kristin Uhler,[15] Karl R White[16] and Mallene Wiggin[1]

[1]University of Colorado, Boulder, Colorado, USA
[2]Global Coalition of Parents of Children who are Deaf or Hard of Hearing (GPODHH), and THRIVE, South Africa
[3]UCL Great Ormond Street Institute of Child Health, London, UK
[4]University of the City of London, London, UK
[5]World Health Organization, Geneva, Switzerland
[6]Ephphatha Listening and Language Center, Taipei, Taiwan
[7]University College London; London School of Economics; Imperial College London; Anglia Ruskin Cambridge, Vision-and-Eye-Research-Institute, UK
[8]University Hospital Münster, Westphalian Wilhelm University, Münster, Germany
[9]Hunter College, City University of New York (CUNY), New York, USA
[10]Institute of Neurology of Senses and Language, Konventhospital Barmherzige Brüder Linz, Linz, Austria
[11]Cincinnati Children's Hospital Medical Center, Cincinnati, Ohio, USA
[12]Pontificia Universidade Católica de São Paulo, São Paulo, Brazil
[13]Great Ormond Street Hospital for Children, London, UK
[14]NextSense Institute, Sydney, Australia
[15]The Children's Hospital Colorado, University of Colorado, Anschutz, Aurora, Colorado, USA
[16]Utah State University, Logan, Utah, USA

Declaration of Independence
This book is as balanced and practical as we can make it.
Ideas for improvement are always welcome: fastfacts@karger.com

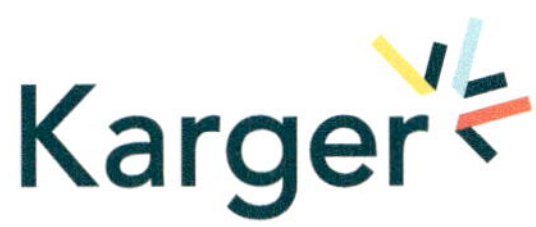

HEALTHCARE

Fast Facts: Early Hearing Detection and Intervention
First published 2023

S. Karger Publishers Ltd, Elizabeth House, Queen Street, Abingdon,
Oxford OX14 3LN, UK
Tel: +44 (0)1235 523233

Book orders can be placed by telephone or email, or via the website.
Please telephone +41 61 306 1440 or email orders@karger.com
To order via the website, please go to karger.com

A CIP record for this title is available from the British Library.

ISBN 978-3-318-06736-1

Yoshinaga-Itano C (Christine)
Fast Facts: Early Hearing Detection and Intervention/
Christine Yoshinaga-Itano

Medical illustrations by Graeme Chambers, Belfast, UK.
Typesetting by Amnet, Chennai, India.
Printed in the UK with Xpedient Print.

List of contributors

Editor

Christine Yoshinaga-Itano PhD
Research Professor, Institute of Cognitive Science
Professor Emerita, Department of Speech, Language & Hearing Sciences
University of Colorado
Boulder, Colorado, USA
Visiting Professor, University of Witwatersrand, South Africa

Contributors

Bianca Birdsey MBChB MSc
Director of Global Family Support Initiatives
Global Coalition of Parents of Children who are Deaf or Hard of Hearing (GPODHH), and Co-founder/Co-director
THRIVE, South Africa

Emma Butcher PhD
UCL Great Ormond Street Institute of Child Health
London, UK

Gwen Carr BA DipEdDeaf FRCA
Honorary Senior Research Associate, and
Independent Consultant
Early Hearing Detection & Intervention
University of the City of London, London, UK

Shelly Chadha MBBS MS PhD
Technical Lead, Ear and Hearing Care Programme
Sensory Functions, Disability, and Rehabilitation Unit
Department for Noncommunicable Diseases
World Health Organization, Geneva, Switzerland

Hsiu-wen Chang PhD
Audiologist and Founder, Ephphatha Listening and Language Center
Taipei, Taiwan

Adrian C Davis OBE PhD HonDFSS FFPH FRSM
Honorary Professor Hearing and Communication
University College, London
Visiting Professor Population Health Science,
London School of Economics
ENT and Audiology, Imperial College, London
Anglia Ruskin Cambridge, Vision-and-Eye-Research-Institute
UK

Harald A Euler PhD
Professor (retired) of Psychology Guest Professor,
Department of Phoniatrics and Pedaudiology
University Hospital Münster
Westphalian Wilhelm University
Münster, Germany

Elaine Gale PhD
Assistant Professor of Deaf and Hard of Hearing,
School of Education
Hunter College
City University of New York (CUNY)
New York, USA

Daniel Holzinger PhD
Head of Centre for Communication and Language
Institute of Neurology of Senses and Language,
Konventhospital Barmherzige Brüder Linz
Linz, Austria

Cynthia Hunnicutt MA
Research Associate, Institute of Cognitive Science
University of Colorado
Boulder, Colorado, USA

Lisa L Hunter PhD
Scientific Director, Audiology
and Professor, Communication Sciences Research Center
Cincinnati Children's Hospital Medical Center
Cincinnati, Ohio, USA

Rachel Knowles MBChB FFPH FRCPCH PhD
Principal Research Fellow
UCL Great Ormond Street Institute of Child Health
London, UK

Doris R Lewis PhD
Professor Titular da PUC-SP, Phonoaudiologia
Pontificia Universidade Católica de São Paulo
São Paulo, Brazil

Vinaya Manchaiah PhD
Professor of Otolaryngology – Head and Neck Surgery
Department of Otolaryngology – Head and Neck Surgery
University of Colorado School of Medicine
Director of Audiology
UCHealth Hearing and Balance
University of Colorado Hospital
Aurora, Colorado, USA

Philipp Mathmann MD
Senior Physician and Deputy Director
Department of Phoniatrics and Pedaudiology
University Hospital Münster
Westphalian Wilhelm University
Münster, Germany

Katrin Neumann MD
Medical Officer WHO Programme for Prevention of Deafness and Hearing Loss
Professor of Population Medicine of Communication Disorders
Director, Department of Phoniatrics and Pedaudiology
University Hospital Münster, Westphalian Wilhelm University
Münster, Germany

Waheeda Pagarkar MRCP MSc
Consultant Audiovestibular Medicine
Great Ormond Street Hospital for Children
London, UK

Allison L Sedey PhD
Director, Outcomes and Developmental Data Assistance
Center for EHDI Programs
University of Colorado
Boulder, Colorado, USA

**Tony KS Sirimanna MBBS DLO(RCS-UK)
FRCS(Ed) FRCP(Hon) MS(Oto) MSc**
Consultant Audiological Physician
Great Ormond Street Hospital for Children (1995–2020)
London, UK

Trudy Smith MA
Manager, Continuing Professional Education
NextSense Institute
Sydney, Australia

Kristin Uhler PhD
Associate Professor, Physical Medicine & Rehabilitation
The Children's Hospital Colorado, University of Colorado
Anschutz Medical Campus, Aurora, Colorado, USA

Karl R White PhD
Founding Director
National Center for Hearing Assessment and Management
Professor of Psychology
Utah State University
Logan, Utah, USA

Mallene Wiggin PhD
Co-Director, Outcomes and Developmental Data Assistance
Center for EHDI Programs
University of Colorado, Boulder, Colorado, USA

List of abbreviations

aABR: automated auditory brainstem response

ABR: auditory brainstem response

ACMG: American College of Medical Genetics and Genomics

AEP: auditory evoked potential

ANSD: auditory neuropathy spectrum disorder

aOAE: automated otoacoustic emission

ASSR: auditory steady-state response

BAHA: bone-anchored hearing aid

BTE: behind the ear

cCMV: congenital cytomegalovirus

CHARGE: coloboma, heart defects, atresia choanae, growth retardation, genital abnormalities and ear abnormalities

CHL: conductive hearing loss

CI: confidence interval

CMV: cytomegalovirus

CNS: central nervous system

CrI: credible interval

CT: computed tomography

dB HL: decibel hearing level

DHH: deaf or hard of hearing

DM: digital modulation

DPOAE: distortion product otoacoustic emission

EHDI: early hearing detection and intervention

FCEI: family-centered early intervention

FDA: (US) Food and Drug Administration

FM: frequency modulation

GDP: gross domestic product

HIV: human immunodeficiency virus

IgG: immunoglobulin G

IPC-EHC: integrated people-centered ear and hearing care

JCIH: Joint Committee on Infant Hearing

MEF: middle ear fluid

MRI: magnetic resonance imaging

NGS: next-generation sequencing

NICHQ: National Institute for Children's Health Quality

NICU: neonatal intensive care unit

NIHS: newborn and infant hearing screening

OAE: otoacoustic emission

PCR: polymerase chain reaction

PHL: permanent hearing loss

RECD: real ear-to-coupler difference

SII: speech intelligibility index

SNHL: sensorineural hearing loss

TEOAE: transient evoked otoacoustic emission

UHL: unilateral hearing loss

UNHS: universal newborn hearing screening

VRA: visual reinforcement audiometry

WES: whole-exome sequencing

WHO: World Health Organization

WIC: women, infant and child

Introduction

There is ample evidence documenting the negative consequences of undiagnosed hearing loss in early childhood. The impact on a child's acquisition of speech, language and literacy and on the development of cognitive and socioemotional skills can be profound, as can the effect on family dynamics. However, despite widespread acceptance of the importance of screening the hearing of newborns and infants, and the existence of the technology that makes this possible, the provision of universal newborn hearing screening (UNHS) programs is not uniform throughout the world.

Moreover, it is a common misconception that simply initiating a UNHS program is sufficient to overcome the impacts of hearing loss. Screening must be supported by access to appropriate diagnostic and early intervention services to support affected children and their families and increase the likelihood of a child achieving age- and cognitively-appropriate development targets. The sooner a child can be screened, diagnosed, fitted with amplification technology and enrolled in early intervention services, the better the outcomes for that child are likely to be. Newborn and infant hearing screening followed by appropriate early intervention has been shown to be effective, cost efficient and an excellent investment of resources.

In *Fast Facts: Early Hearing Detection and Intervention* an international team of contributors brings together the evidence that supports the effectiveness of UNHS and early hearing detection and intervention services (EHDI). As well as considering elements essential to successful UNHS/EHDI programs, including screening technologies, resources, data management and family-centered early intervention services, the team discusses the resources needed to deliver such programs as well as the performance of screening programs globally. The aim is to provide a comprehensive compendium of information to make the case for greater recognition of the importance of UNHS/EHDI and so improve the life chances of children who are diagnosed as deaf or hard of hearing.

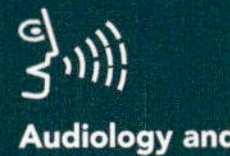

Audiology and Speech

—

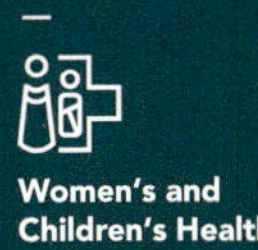

Women's and Children's Health

1 Newborn hearing screening and EHDI

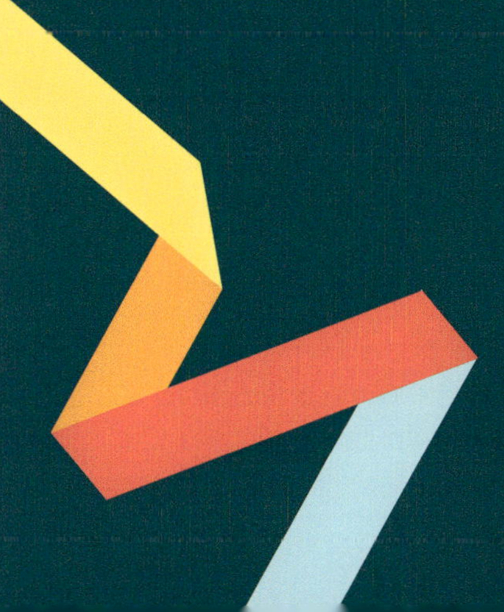

HEALTHCARE

The consequences of undiagnosed hearing loss in early childhood can be significant, with negative impacts on a child's language, cognitive and socioemotional development, as well as on their literacy and vocational potential. The effect on the family of an affected child can also be profound. As a result, children with hearing loss are at high risk of requiring specialized education and experiencing difficulty or an inability to function in society without support.

Early hearing detection and intervention (EHDI) programs can help alleviate the negative consequences of childhood hearing loss. Universal newborn hearing screening (UNHS)/EHDI programs have been established in many high-income countries, but are less common in low- and middle-income countries.

Screening technologies

It has been possible to screen the hearing of newborn babies within the first few days of life since the early 1990s. Two different technologies are used to conduct neonatal hearing screening (Figure 1.1).

Automated otoacoustic emission (aOAE) screening uses automated technology to assess the function of the outer hair cells in the cochlear while a newborn baby or a child is lying still, either in natural sleep or with mild sedation. A probe containing a microphone is placed in the ear canal, clicks or pure tones are sent through it and a machine measures the type of echo the sound causes in the outer hair cells. aOAE testing is unable to detect hearing loss resulting from issues beyond the outer hair cells in the auditory pathway, for example, auditory neuropathy spectrum disorder (ANSD) where the lesion occurs somewhere in the auditory nerve.

Automated auditory brainstem response (aABR) screening measures whether the auditory nerve transmits sound from the inner ear to the brainstem, and how loud sounds have to be for the brain to detect them. This automated test can indicate if the brain is not receiving the information in a clear way. aABR screening is conducted while the infant is asleep, preferably in natural sleep. Electrodes are placed on the child's head to measure brain activity and the sound is presented either through earphones or a probe placed into the ear canal.

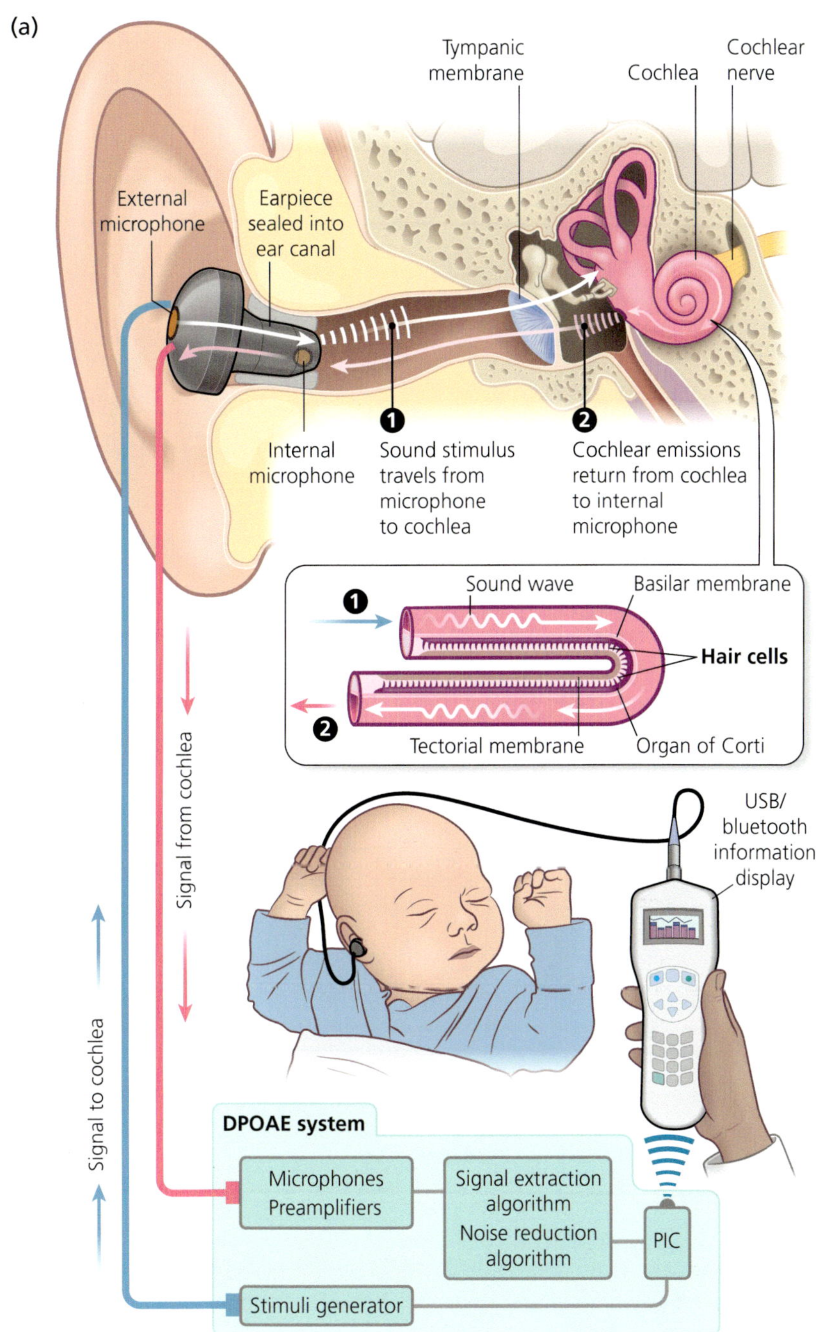
(a)
Tympanic membrane
Cochlea
Cochlear nerve
External microphone
Earpiece sealed into ear canal
Internal microphone
1 Sound stimulus travels from microphone to cochlea
2 Cochlear emissions return from cochlea to internal microphone
Sound wave
Basilar membrane
Hair cells
Tectorial membrane
Organ of Corti
Signal from cochlea
Signal to cochlea
USB/ bluetooth information display
DPOAE system
Microphones Preamplifiers
Signal extraction algorithm
Noise reduction algorithm
PIC
Stimuli generator

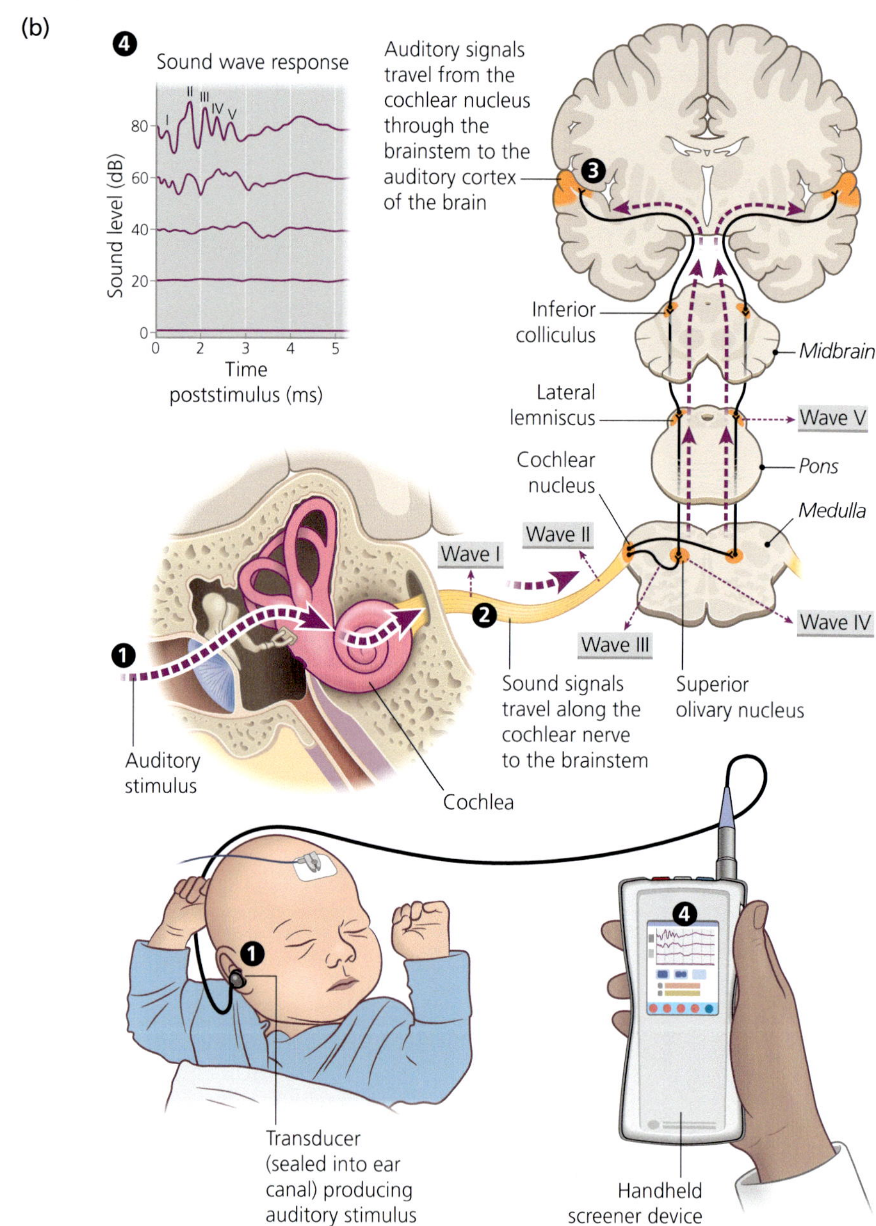

Figure 1.1 Newborn infants undergoing (a) aOAE and (b) aABR screening.

The hearing screen is typically completed in 1–4 minutes per ear. Many newborn hearing screening programs use both aOAE and aABR to test a baby's hearing, although some programs use one type of testing only. Because the screening tests are not 100% accurate, if families suspect that their child is not hearing well, even if newborn screening was not suggestive of hearing loss, they should be referred for further testing.

Diagnostic audiological evaluations for confirmation of hearing loss after newborn hearing screening include diagnostic ABR and OAE testing and are discussed in more detail in Chapter 10.

Integrated systems

Although technology provides a means of screening all newborns shortly after birth, newborn hearing screening itself represents only the first step in a complex EHDI system and care pathway. High-quality EHDI programs have been successfully established and implemented in many countries throughout the world but integrating such programs with timely enrollment into early intervention services has not been as successful, increasing the likelihood that children who are deaf or hard of hearing (DHH) may not achieve age- or cognitively-appropriate development targets.

A high-quality integrated EHDI program should aim to achieve the EHDI 1–3–6 benchmarks set by the Joint Committee on Infant Hearing (JCIH): screen by 1 month, identify by 3 months and enroll into early intervention services by 6 months. Ideally, where resources allow, the benchmarks should be 1–2–3, with screening by 1 month, identification by 2 months and enrollment in early intervention by 3 months.

The EHDI model illustrated in Figure 1.2 represents an integrated system, with all elements being core to achieving successful outcomes for a child and their family. All high-quality systems should be underpinned by the following key principles.

- Infants who are referred after newborn hearing screening should receive timely audiological and medical assessment and management, using best practices in assessment and diagnosis.

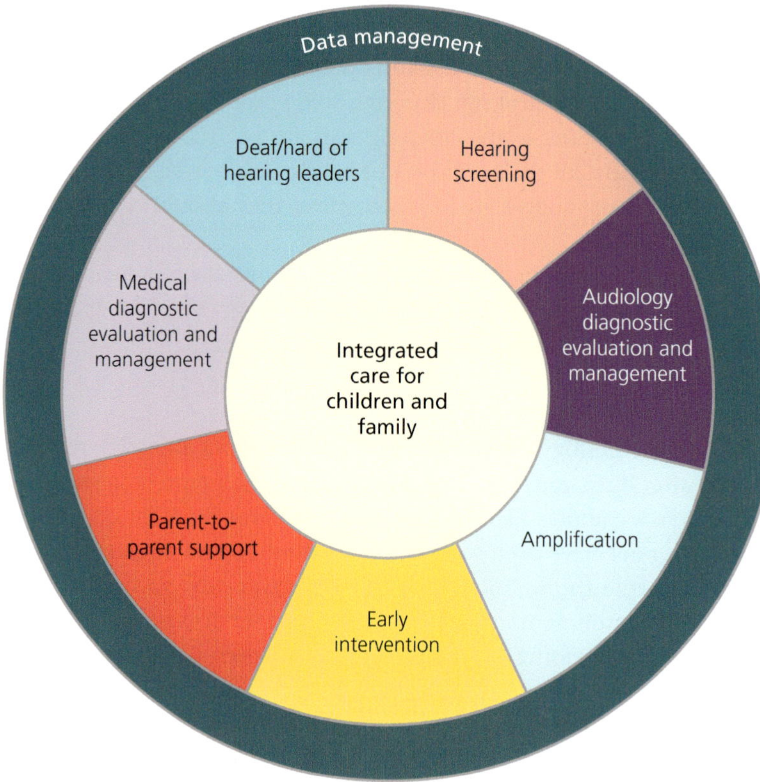

Figure 1.2 Elements of an integrated EHDI system.

- With parental agreement, infants should be provided with appropriately fitted amplification and be referred for cochlear implantation when they meet both audiological criteria and national candidacy criteria (see Chapter 11).
- Skilled support should be available for families and for the assessment and promotion of spoken and/or visual language, speech and/or sign phonology, language (spoken/signed), communication and socioemotional development in young children, following confirmation of hearing loss.

- Accurate and effective data capture and management systems (discussed in greater detail in Chapter 8) should enable quality assurance of the program and effective tracking throughout the full pathway, including tracking the longitudinal developmental milestones of identified children.
- All personnel delivering the services should have appropriate skills and competencies and access to training and ongoing professional development.
- Parents and professionals who are DHH should be fully involved in strategic planning and at all levels of program delivery.
- There should be a good flow of communication across the pathway that promotes effective management by professionals and a coordinated experience for families.

Key points – newborn hearing screening and early hearing detection and intervention

- Integrated EHDI systems can help alleviate the negative consequences of congenital or early childhood hearing loss.
- Newborn hearing testing is only the first step of a complex EHDI system.
- Two technologies are used to screen hearing in newborn babies, aOAE testing and aABR testing.
- Comprehensive integrated EHDI systems aim to meet the 1–3–6 benchmarks, namely that all infants are screened for hearing loss by 1 month of age, affected infants are identified by 3 months and are enrolled into early intervention/therapeutic services by 6 months. When EHDI 1–3–6 has been accomplished, systems should strive for 1–2–3 benchmarks (screen by 1 month, identify by 2 months and enroll in intervention by 3 months).

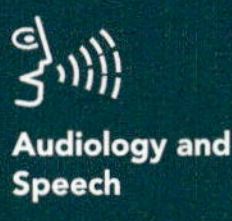

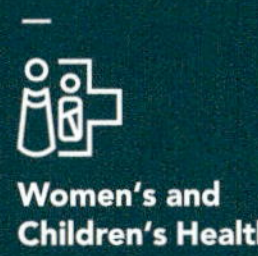

2 Rationale for UNHS/EHDI programs

Christine Yoshinaga-Itano, Vinaya Manchaiah and Cynthia Hunnicutt

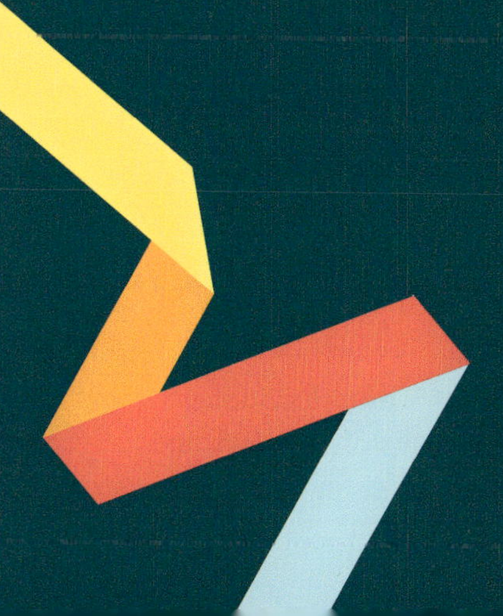

HEALTHCARE

Efficacy of UNHS/EHDI programs

Achieving optimal developmental outcomes depends not only on early identification of hearing loss but also on early access to therapeutic intervention services and to amplification. However, to convince government agencies, hospitals and insurance companies that it is worthwhile investing money in establishing UNHS/EHDI programs, it is critical to demonstrate that such programs are efficacious.

Identification of hearing loss. All studies of UNHS/EHDI have found that hearing loss is identified at a significantly younger age (1–9 months versus 2 years or older) in children exposed to UNHS/EHDI programs than in those with no exposure to UNHS/EHDI programs.[1–5]

Amplification device fitting is achieved earlier in children with hearing loss who have access to UNHS/EHDI than in those who do not (2.7–13.5 months versus 24.0–29.1 months).[2,3,6,7]

Initiation of early intervention services begins at a younger age (2.5–8.9 months) in children with hearing loss who are exposed to UNHS/EHDI than in those who are not (30.5 months).[6]

Language development. Language levels within the expected range have been reported through to the age of 5 years for children with hearing loss after UNHS/EHDI exposure in the USA in contrast to significantly delayed receptive and expressive language among children not exposed to UNHS/EHDI.[4,5,8] Children meeting the EHDI 1–3–6 benchmarks (see Chapter 1) have significantly higher language levels than those who do not meet the 1–3–6 benchmarks, even if they have been screened for hearing loss as newborns (Figure 2.1).[9]

Poorer language and reading skills in middle childhood (mean age 7.9 years) have been shown to increase the risk of teacher-rated problem behaviors and socioemotional difficulties.[10–12] Children in these studies tended not to meet the EHDI 1–3–6 benchmarks.

UNHS versus distraction hearing screening at 9 months. Studies in the UK have found that children who were exposed to UNHS, and

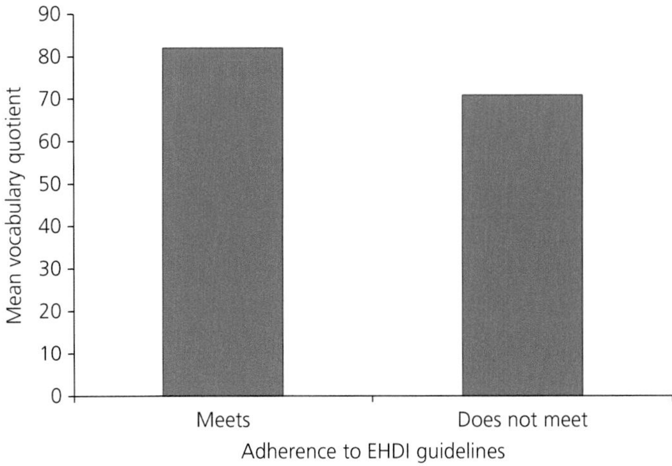

Figure 2.1 Mean vocabulary quotients for children meeting the 1–3–6 EHDI guidelines versus those who did not meet the EHDI guidelines.

those whose hearing loss was identified by the age of 9 months, had significantly better language and reading skills by 6–9 years of age than those who were exposed to distraction hearing screening at the age of 9 months.[13,14] One study reported that identifying hearing loss in children before the age of 9 months (regardless of the method of detection) also predicted significantly better reading outcomes between 12 and 19 years of age when compared with children whose hearing loss was identified after 9 months of age.[14]

In Australia, exposure to UNHS predicted better language scores for children at 3–5 years of age when compared against distraction hearing screening or opportunistic identification,[2] while in the Netherlands, children who were exposed to UNHS as opposed to distraction screening were found to have better social development and quality of life at 3–5 years of age.[15]

In the USA, children aged 3–5 years had better speech production and speech perception after exposure to UNHS.[5,6] However, a UK study found that speech production did not differ significantly between children who were exposed to UNHS or early confirmation of hearing loss (mean age of identification by 9 months) and those who were not.[1]

Impact on families. There have been a number of studies into the impact of UNHS on the families of children being screened. These have found no evidence of negative effects such as greater levels of anxiety, stress or depression among:

- mothers whose infants participated in UNHS/EHDI programs when compared with mothers whose infants did not[16–18]
- families with infants with negative versus positive screening results[19,20]
- families with positive findings after the first versus the second screen[21,22]
- families with anxiety about UNHS versus other maternal anxieties.[23,24]

Long-term outcomes. At present, little is known about long-term outcomes in the areas of auditory development and speech production for children exposed to UNHS/EHDI as compared with those who were not. Also unknown is the long-term impact of exposure on problem behaviors, quality of life and socioemotional development.

Creating effective UNHS/EHDI systems

It is a common misconception that simply instituting a newborn hearing screening program will result in optimal outcomes for children with early childhood hearing loss. In fact, developing effective UNHS/EDHI programs requires a focus not only on implementing screening of newborns, but also on investment in diagnostic evaluation facilities and quality early intervention therapeutic services. Unless pediatric audiological diagnostic facilities staffed by personnel trained in infant diagnosis and following evidence-based protocols are available and accessible, timely identification of hearing loss will still not occur.

Likewise, access to early intervention therapeutic services is equally important to justify the expense of establishing UNHS/EHDI systems. Without habilitative, educational support services for families who have newly diagnosed infants, optimal developmental outcomes are less likely to be achieved.

Meeting all of the EHDI 1–3–6 benchmarks is critical for optimal vocabulary development and better pragmatic language skills in children who are DHH. Failure to meet either the second (identification by 3 months) or third (in early intervention services by 6 months) benchmarks after implementing UNHS has been found to be comparable to missing both benchmarks.[9]

Key points – rationale for UNHS/EHDI programs

- Effective UNHS/EHDI programs lead to earlier identification of hearing loss and earlier access to both therapeutic intervention services and amplification.
- Children whose hearing loss is identified before the age of 9 months show better language and reading skills later in childhood than children who are older when their hearing loss is identified.
- A hearing screening program alone is insufficient to achieve optimal development outcomes for children with early childhood hearing loss.

References

1. Kennedy CR, McCann DC, Campbell MJ et al. Language ability after early detection of permanent childhood hearing impairment. *N Engl J Med* 2006;354:2131–41.
2. Wake M, Ching TY, Wirth K et al. Population outcomes of three approaches to detection of congenital hearing loss. *Pediatrics* 2016;137:e20151722.
3. Wood SA, Sutton GJ, Davis A. Performance and characteristics of the Newborn Hearing Screening Programme in England: the first seven years. *Int J Audiol* 2015;54:353–8.
4. Yoshinaga-Itano C, Sedey A, Coulter DK, Mehl AL. Language of early- and later-identified children with hearing loss. *Pediatrics* 1998;102:1161–71.
5. Yoshinaga-Itano C, Coulter D, Thomson V. The Colorado Newborn Hearing Screening Project: effects on speech and language development for children with hearing loss. *J Perinatol* 2000;20:S131–6.
6. Sininger YS, Martinez A, Eisenberg L et al. Newborn hearing screening speeds diagnosis and access to intervention by 20–25 months. *J Am Acad Audiol* 2009;20:49–57.

7. Uus K, Bamford J. Effectiveness of population-based newborn hearing screening in England: ages of interventions and profile of cases. *Pediatrics* 2006;117:e887–93.
8. Yoshinaga-Itano C, Coulter D, Thomson V. Developmental outcomes of children with hearing loss born in Colorado hospitals with and without universal newborn hearing screening programs. *Semin Neonatol* 2001;6:521–9.
9. Yoshinaga-Itano C, Sedey AL, Wiggin M, Chung C. Early hearing detection and vocabulary of children with hearing loss. *Pediatrics* 2017;140:e20162964.
10. Stevenson J, McCann DC, Law CM et al. The effect of early confirmation of hearing loss on the behavior in middle childhood of children with bilateral hearing impairment. *Dev Med Child Neurol* 2011; 53:269–74.
11. Stevenson J, Kreppner J, Pimperton H et al. Emotional and behavioural difficulties in children and adolescents with hearing impairment: a systematic review and meta-analysis. *Eur Child Adolesc Psychiatry* 2015;24:477–96.
12. Stevenson J, McCann D, Watkin P et al. The relationship between language development and behaviour problems in children with hearing loss. *J Child Psychol Psychiatry* 2010;51:77–83.
13. McCann DC, Worsfold S, Law CM et al. Reading and communication skills after universal newborn hearing screening for permanent childhood hearing impairment. *Arch Dis Child* 2009;94:293–7.
14. Pimperton H, Blythe H, Kreppner J et al. The impact of universal newborn hearing screening on long-term literacy outcomes: a prospective cohort study. *Arch Dis Child* 2016;101:9–15.
15. Korver AM, Konings S, Dekker FW et al; DECIBEL Collaborative Study Group. Newborn hearing screening vs later hearing screening and developmental outcomes in children with permanent childhood hearing impairment. *JAMA* 2010;304:1701–8.
16. Watkin PM, Baldwin M, Dixon R, Beckman A. Maternal anxiety and attitudes to universal neonatal hearing screening. *Br J Audiol* 1998; 32:27–37.
17. Crockett R, Wright AJ, Uus K et al. Maternal anxiety following newborn hearing screening: the moderating role of knowledge. *J Med Screen* 2006;13:20–5.
18. Crockett R, Marteau T, Uus K et al. Maternal anxiety and satisfaction following infant hearing screening: a comparison of the health visitor distraction test and newborn hearing screening. *J Med Screen* 2005;12:78–82.

19. Wessex Universal Neonatal Hearing Screening Trial Group. Controlled trial of universal neonatal screening for early identification of permanent childhood hearing impairment. *Lancet* 1998;352:1957–64.
20. Stuart A, Moretz M, Yang EY. An investigation of maternal stress after neonatal hearing screening. *Am J Audiol* 2000;9:135–41.
21. Vohr BR, Letourneau KS, McDermott C. Maternal worry about neonatal hearing screening. *J Perinatol* 2001;21:15–20.
22. Weichbold V, Welzl-Mueller K. Maternal concern about positive test results in universal newborn hearing screening. *Pediatrics* 2001;108:1111–16.
23. Tueller SJ. Maternal worry about infant health, maternal anxiety, and maternal perceptions of child vulnerability associated with newborn hearing screening results. Master's thesis (unpublished), Logan: Utah State University, 2006.
24. Tueller SJ, White KR. Maternal anxiety associated with newborn hearing screening. *J Early Hear Detect Interv* 2016;1:87–92.

Further reading and resources

Family-Centered Early Intervention International. FCEI principles. www.fcei.at/unit/fcei/positionstatement/fcei

Joint Committee on Infant Hearing. Position statements. www.jcih.org/posstatemts.htm

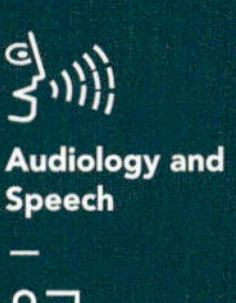

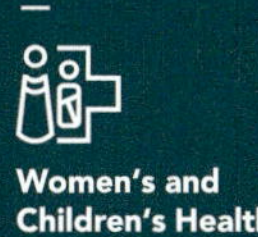

3 Prevalence of newborn hearing loss and performance of screening programs

Emma Butcher and Rachel Knowles

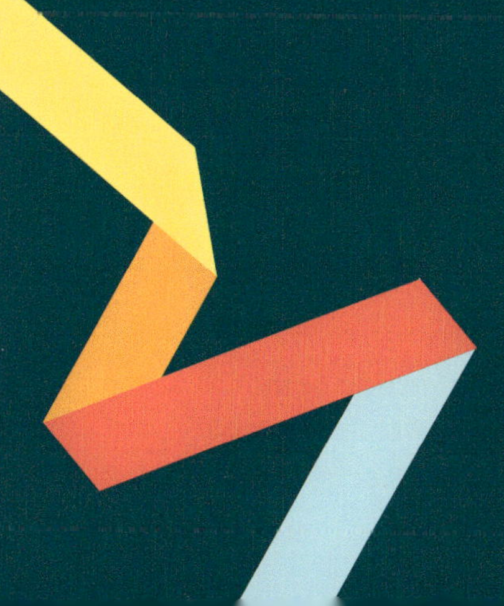

HEALTHCARE

Hearing loss is the most common sensory deficit in the world, affecting more than 250 million people.[1] Many countries have introduced UNHS but programs vary in how they are implemented and how they perform. Understanding these variations is key to improving the early detection, diagnosis and clinical management of hearing loss in children.[2,3]

Prevalence

The existence of UNHS in a country influences the reported prevalence of hearing loss in contemporary screened populations. Knowing the prevalence of hearing loss at birth is essential to inform planning for the healthcare, educational and other relevant services that will be required by newborns and young children with hearing loss, as well as for examining UNHS performance in terms of sensitivity, specificity and cost-effectiveness.

Two systematic reviews have synthesized information on the prevalence of permanent hearing loss (PHL) (hearing loss of ≥40 dB) detected through screening in the first year of life. The first review, by Butcher et al. (2019),[4] included very highly developed countries and limited the case definition to bilateral hearing loss. It reported a prevalence estimate for hearing loss of 1.2 (95% confidence interval [CI] 1.0, 1.4) per 1000 screened infants.[4]

A similar prevalence estimate for bilateral hearing loss of 1.3 (credible interval [CrI] 1.0, 1.6) per 1000 children was reported in the second review by Bussé et al. (2020).[5] This review used data on bilateral and unilateral hearing loss (UHL) identified in screening programs and audiometric studies from low- to high-income countries. It also reported an estimated prevalence of UHL of 0.8 (CrI 0.5, 1.1) per 1000 children and an estimated prevalence of UHL and bilateral hearing loss combined of approximately 2.2 (CrI 1.7, 2.8) per 1000 children.[5]

Both meta-analyses identified high variability in detected prevalence across individual studies. This was likely due to differences in the detection methods used and the ability to exclude temporary hearing loss.[4,5]

Regional variation. Both reviews identified differences in the prevalence of hearing loss by location. The first analysis reported a lower prevalence in Australia than in Europe, Asia and North America.[4] The second analysis found no significant differences in prevalence by region or gross national income per capita; however, the highest prevalences were found in Nigeria, India, Hong Kong and Iran and the lowest prevalences were detected in Ireland, South Africa, Brazil and China.[5] It seems clear that regional differences in prevalence do exist. These may be explained by the distribution of genetic and environmental risk factors. Further research is required to confirm which areas have higher prevalence and to fully investigate the explanatory factors.

Intensive care admission. Admission to a neonatal intensive care unit (NICU) is a known risk factor for hearing loss. Both reviews identified a five to eight times higher prevalence of hearing loss among infants who were admitted to a NICU than among those who were not.

More specifically, Butcher et al. identified a prevalence of bilateral hearing loss of 5.1 (95% CI 2.5, 5.8) per 1000 screened infants admitted to a NICU compared with 0.9 (95% CI 0.5, 1.4) per 1000 screened infants in the well-baby population.[4] Bussé et al. identified a prevalence of bilateral and unilateral PHL of 15.8 (CrI 4.7, 29.5) per 1000 children among those admitted to a NICU compared with 1.9 (CrI 1.1, 3.0) per 1000 children in the well-baby population.[5]

Evaluating UNHS program performance

UNHS most often takes place in a hospital and is completed by trained medical professionals. Screening in the first few days of life is preferred, especially in settings where in-hospital births are common.[6] In the meta-analysis by Butcher et al., UNHS performance was good across all of the included studies (in Europe, North America and Australia).[4] The sensitivity (detection rate) for bilateral hearing loss was high (89–100%), as was screening specificity (92–100%). The negative predictive value, reflecting the accuracy of screening in correctly identifying newborns with normal hearing, was 100% across the studies that identified false-negative screening results (that is, children who passed screening but were later diagnosed with hearing loss).

These findings must be interpreted cautiously as most studies of UNHS programs did not follow up children with screen-negative results and therefore may have missed cases of hearing loss. In the few studies that did follow up these children, robust monitoring methods were not always used, meaning that false-negative cases, as well as children with later-onset or progressive hearing loss, may not have been detected.[4]

Positive predictive value. To effectively evaluate screening program performance, children with screen-positive results should be followed up until hearing status is confirmed. This allows estimation of the proportion of positive screen results that accurately identify true cases of bilateral hearing loss, known as the positive predictive value.

In the meta-analysis by Butcher et al., positive predictive values reported by different studies of UNHS varied markedly from 2–84%.[4] Programs that achieve only low positive predictive values should institute measures to reduce the number of false positives and avoid the potential for parental distress and over-investigation that can arise from false-positive test results.[5] Assessing the reasons for poor performance, such as high loss to follow-up, is key.

Testing protocols. The performance of UNHS programs is also determined by the type of testing and the test protocols used. There is a lack of consensus about best practice in terms of protocols or screening instruments, leading to significant variation between current UNHS programs with regard to the number and order of testing stages. In the meta-analysis by Butcher et al.:

- a combination of OAE and ABR testing was used in 54% of included programs
- OAE testing only was reported in 26% of programs and ABR testing only was reported in 20% of programs.[4]

OAE testing is common as the initial test in many UNHS programs because it is simple and relatively low cost. Repeated OAE tests at different time points, or repeat testing at a single time point, increases screening specificity versus a single OAE test.[7]

The ABR screening test has a higher sensitivity and specificity than OAE. ABR also identifies certain conditions that OAE testing cannot, such as ANSD; however, ABR testing is usually more expensive than

OAE testing and is more difficult to use in out-of-hospital settings. It is therefore often used in the later stages of screening programs and in a hospital or clinic environment.[7]

Different screening protocols are employed for children with specific risk factors for hearing loss, often reducing the number of testing stages or using ABR earlier in the screening pathway. The number of screening stages in the meta-analysis by Butcher et al. ranged from one to five, although most programs used two or three stages before diagnostic referral.[4]

Cost-effectiveness

Screening an entire newborn population is expensive; therefore, cost must be carefully considered in UNHS programs. In a health technology assessment, the estimated costs per detected infant with hearing loss were €10 306 for UNHS, €2592 for selective screening and €1402 without systematic screening.[8] These estimates depended on the cost, specificity and sensitivity of individual tests and on screening program coverage. The costs of UNHS were deemed reasonable because UNHS is more effective in detecting hearing loss than other strategies and will provide long-term benefits, including productivity benefits arising from improved language skills achieved following early intervention. Additionally, the costs are similar to those of other screening programs. Further economic evaluations across a wide range of settings and with varied methodologies have also concluded that UNHS is cost-effective.[8]

Future economic evaluations should focus on improving the measurement of utility and long-term costs and benefits, as well as carrying out comprehensive sensitivity analyses (for instance comparing different ages at screening, and differences in screening coverage).[9] This could identify factors that would improve the performance of UNHS programs, such as the optimal number of stages in the screening protocol or the use of OAE versus ABR tests at each stage.

Improving the performance of UNHS programs

Population-based programs with good coverage and follow-up are likely to bring the greatest benefits in detecting hearing loss. However, one study has found that around 20% of newborns are lost to follow-up after UNHS. Addressing barriers such as travel costs and lack of parental awareness of the importance of follow-up, and strengthening monitoring systems, could improve follow-up rates in screening programs where they are poor.[10]

A balance must be struck in optimizing the performance of UNHS programs. For instance, the use of multiple testing stages increases resource use and the burden of attendance but can also increase screening performance and reduce referrals for diagnostic tests.[11] UNHS protocols must consider the target conditions that they are screening for (which can vary from permanent, bilateral and severe hearing loss to temporary, unilateral or mild hearing loss), the timing of tests and the level of outcome monitoring appropriate for the population and healthcare system in which screening is being implemented.

Key points – prevalence of newborn hearing loss and performance of screening programs

- Knowing the prevalence of hearing loss among newborns and young children informs planning for healthcare, educational and other services for those affected.
- Two separate reviews have reported prevalence estimates for bilateral hearing loss of 1.2 and 1.3 per 1000 screened infants, respectively.
- There appears to be regional variation in the prevalence of hearing loss; this may reflect the distribution of genetic and environmental risk factors.
- The types of test used and the testing protocols followed influence the performance of UNHS programs.
- UNHS is more effective than other screening strategies in identifying hearing loss in newborns and offers associated long-term benefits, including productivity benefits arising from improved language skills achieved through early intervention.

References

1. Mathers C, Smith A, Concha M. Global burden of hearing loss in the year 2000. *Global Burden of Disease 2000*, vol 18. Geneva: World Health Organization, 2000. www.who.int/healthinfo/statistics/bod_hearingloss.pdf, last accessed 4 November 2021.
2. Yoshinaga-Itano C, Sedey AL, Coulter DK, Mehl AL. Language of early- and later-identified children with hearing loss. *Pediatrics* 1998;102:1161–71.
3. Kennedy CR, McCann DC, Campbell MJ et al. Language ability after early detection of permanent childhood hearing impairment. *N Engl J Med* 2006;354:2131–41.
4. Butcher E, Dezateux C, Cortina-Borja M, Knowles RL. Prevalence of permanent childhood hearing loss detected at the universal newborn hearing screen: systematic review and meta-analysis. *PLoS One* 2019;14:e0219600.
5. Bussé AM, Hoeve HL, Nasserinejad K et al. Prevalence of permanent neonatal hearing impairment: systematic review and Bayesian meta-analysis. *Int J Audiol* 2020;59:475–85
6. Vos B, Senterre C, Lagasse R et al. Organisation of newborn hearing screening programmes in the European Union: widely implemented, differently performed. *Eur J Public Health* 2016;26:505–10.
7. Kanji A, Khoza-Shangase K, Moroe N. Newborn hearing screening protocols and their outcomes: a systematic review. *Int J Pediatr Otorhinolaryngol* 2018;115:104–9.
8. Schnell-Inderst P, Kunze S, Hessel F et al. Screening of the hearing of newborns – update. *GMS Health Technol Assess* 2006;2:Doc20.
9. Sharma R, Gu Y, Ching TY et al. Economic evaluations of childhood hearing loss screening programmes: a systematic review and critique. *Appl Health Econ Health Policy* 2019;15:331–57.
10. Ravi R, Gunjawate DR, Yerraguntla K et al. Follow-up in newborn hearing screening – a systematic review. *Int J Pediatr Otorhinolaryngol* 2016;90:29–36.
11. Clemens CJ, Davis SA. Minimizing false-positives in universal newborn hearing screening: a simple solution. *Pediatrics* 2001;107:e29.

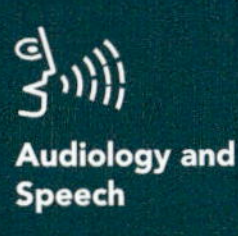

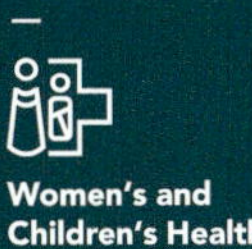

4 Global status of newborn and infant hearing screening

Katrin Neumann, Harald A Euler,
Philipp Mathmann, Shelly Chadha
and Karl R White

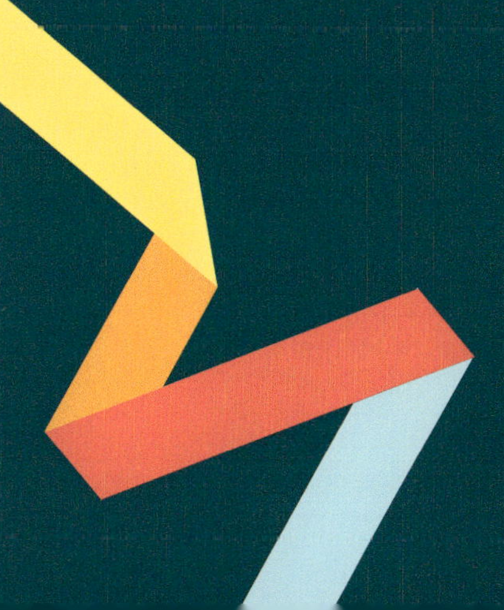

HEALTHCARE

Un- or undertreated hearing loss imposes a significant burden on affected individuals, especially when it starts early in life.[1] As discussed in Chapter 1, PHL in childhood is associated with deficits in language, cognitive, psychosocial and academic development, as well as with negative consequences for employment and earnings.[1,2] There is ample short- and long-term evidence that newborn and infant hearing screening (NIHS) significantly reduces the age of diagnosis and intervention in cases of PHL and improves language, cognitive, socioemotional, academic and professional outcomes in infants who receive timely and suitable care.[3–9]

The cost-effectiveness of NIHS has also been demonstrated.[1,5,10,11] UNHS and measures to prevent hearing loss are most effective in reducing the prevalence of PHL and its sequelae, with UNHS being very effective for high-income countries, and prevention measures expected to show higher relative effects for low-income countries.[12]

In 1995, the WHO adopted a resolution urging member states to prepare national plans for the prevention and control of major causes of avoidable hearing loss, and for early detection of hearing loss in babies, toddlers and children.[13] However, by 2012, only 32 countries had reported the implementation of such policies, and the WHO highlighted a scarcity of epidemiological and other data regarding ear and hearing care.[14] A second WHO resolution, adopted in 2017, reaffirmed the aims of the first and called on member states to collect high-quality population-based data on hearing loss and ear diseases.[15]

Consistent with this goal, and to serve as a baseline for further improving the effectiveness of NIHS, a survey of the global status of NIHS program coverage, strategies and outcomes, as well as the relationship between national economic indices and key screening metrics, has been conducted.[16] In response to the 2017 resolution, the WHO released the first *World Report on Hearing* in March 2021.[1] This summarizes epidemiological and financial data on hearing loss around the world and proposes cost-effective solutions for achieving 'integrated people-centered ear and hearing care' (IPC-EHC). The report recognizes NIHS as playing a key role in IPC-EHC by identifying 'effective coverage of newborn hearing screening services within the population' (the proportion of infants with

PHL who have received appropriate interventions within the first 6 months of life) as one of three tracer indicators for global surveillance and monitoring of progress in ear and hearing care.[1]

Global status of NIHS

The *World Report on Hearing* also refers to the NIHS global status survey mentioned above.[16] This survey includes country-specific information from 158 countries and independent territories (which will be referred to as countries in this chapter). Data for the survey were collected between 2013 and 2019 from respondents at ministries of health, non-governmental organizations and professionals involved in early identification of PHL. The survey results are a good reflection of the global situation, as the participating countries represent almost 95% of the world's population.[16]

NIHS program coverage. According to the survey, less than one-third of the world's population had access to NIHS programs that covered at least 85% of all babies, despite evidence of the effectiveness of this strategy for optimal rehabilitation of children who are DHH. About 38% of countries had no or minimal NIHS (less than 1% coverage) (Figure 4.1).

The prevalence of PHL in children identified through NIHS programs ranged from 0.3–15.0 per 1000 infants with a median of 1.70, according to the survey results.[16] This figure approaches WHO prevalence estimates of 2 per 1000 for the neonatal period.[1]

Age at diagnosis and intervention. Encouragingly, the survey indicated that infants with PHL who underwent NIHS were diagnosed at an average age of 4.6 months and began intervention on average at 6.7 months, an age that falls within the sensitive time windows of auditory pathway maturation when brain structures are physiologically amenable to treatment.[17] This was not true for non-screened children, for whom hearing loss was identified on average at 34.9 months and who did not receive initial intervention until 36.7 months of age.

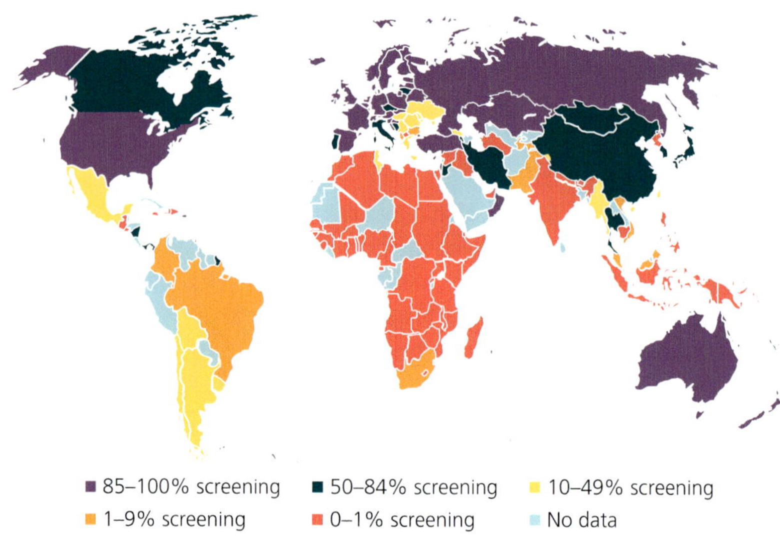

Figure 4.1 Country-specific coverage of NIHS programs. Reproduced with permission from Neumann et al. 2020.[16]

Screening. According to the survey, most NIHS programs use 'physiological' (objective) screening methods. These include OAE measurements to assess inner ear function, aABR recordings to evaluate auditory pathway function up to the brainstem and two-stage OAE-aABR procedures in which aABR is recorded only when OAE fails. These methods achieve high validity, in contrast to behavioral or questionnaire-based methods.[18] Of the infants screened with these standard methods in a reference year, 66.5% were screened with OAE alone, 14.3% with aABR alone and 19.2% with an OAE-aABR combination. Only six countries reported using behavioral methods, and maternal questionnaires or tympanometry were rarely employed. OAE was the preferred method in 57% of countries, followed by OAE-aABR (30%) and aABR (11%).[16]

Screening was performed in birth facilities in 93% of the countries, in other places such as pediatric, hearing care, immunization or well-baby clinics in 51%, and in homes in 14% (the percentages sum to more than 100% because screening could be performed in multiple places within a single country). It was carried out by physicians (26%

of the countries), audiologists or audiological staff (69%), technicians (16%), nurses and midwives (69%), and non-professionals such as community health workers (24%).[16]

Children lost to follow-up. On average, 4.5% of the babies who underwent NIHS failed the screening. The proportion of infants failing screening was significantly lower in countries with NIHS coverage of 85% or more and its range was narrower (0.3–11.6%) compared with countries with lower screening coverage. Of particular concern are the reported 17.2% of children who failed screening but were lost to follow-up. These rates were 8% lower in countries with high NIHS coverage than in countries with low coverage.[16]

A lack of systematic data collection and databases compromises the quality of many screening programs. Accordingly, the tracking of babies who do not receive screening and those who fail screening and need referral to audiological diagnostic and treatment services is poor in many countries. Without tracking, the lost-to-follow-up rate is generally high or simply unknown. Of the countries that reported trustworthy lost-to-follow-up rates, 48%[16] were above the 30% criterion recommended by the JCIH,[19] confirming the results of a meta-analysis which identified lost-to-follow-up rates of more than 30% in many of the studies it analyzed,[20] and implying that nearly one-half of NIHS programs are losing too many children with suspected hearing loss before diagnosis.

High lost-to-follow-up rates have been attributed to a lack of data collection and tracking systems, a lack of audiology services, distance and transportation difficulties, parental anxiety, insecurity, educational disparities and a lack of knowledge about hearing loss. Suitable data management systems have been reported as the most commonly used strategy to overcome these difficulties.[21,22]

Living standards. It is striking that screening coverage and other measures are closely associated with average living standards, as measured by national average nominal gross domestic product per capita (GDP; Table 4.1). Countries with NIHS coverage of 85% or more have median living standards that are 10 times higher than those in countries with screening coverage of less than 10%. However, while countries without hearing screening or with coverage of less than 1%

TABLE 4.1

Global coverage of newborn and infant hearing screening

Coverage of screening	Number of countries	Percentage of countries	Percentage of world population*	GDP (nominal) per capita, average
0%–<1%	64	32.7	37.63	3.7
1%–9%	14	7.1	7.42	3.9
10%–49%	19	9.7	8.33	10.7
50%–84%	17	8.7	6.72	14.4
85%–100%	41	20.9	32.59	40.4
No/insufficient data	41	20.9	6.09	8.6
Total	196	100	98.78	

*The entries do not add up to exactly 100% because of unlisted dependent and disrupted territories. Reproduced with permission from Neumann et al. 2020.[16]

tend to have low living standards, countries with coverage of 85% or more have a large variance in GDP and include countries with low GDP (<10) such as Belarus, China, Kazakhstan, Marshall Islands, Micronesia and Russia.

GDP correlates negatively with screening failure rate, prevalence of PHL, median age at diagnosis and median age at intervention onset. The dramatically lower standard of living in countries with low screening coverage is all the more significant given that 80% of people with disabling hearing loss live in low- and middle-income countries,[23] where poor birth conditions and a lack of vaccination programs contribute significantly to the incidence of PHL,[24] and global production of hearing aids meets less than 3% of the needs of these countries.[22]

NIHS programs with coverage of 85% or more have been initiated in countries such as the USA, Uruguay, most European countries, Israel, Kazakhstan, Oman, Qatar, South Korea, the Seychelles, Australia, New Zealand and the Pacific Island nations that are territories of the USA. Other countries, such as Canada, Mongolia, Panama and China, have implemented large-scale NIHS programs, although they are not nationwide. Interestingly, these countries are by no means all high-income countries. Thus, implementation of NIHS programs appears to depend not only on national wealth, but also on factors such as awareness and attention to infant hearing health among a country's policymakers and health professionals. This is also consistent with the finding that although national mandates are associated with screening coverage (Spearman's $\rho=0.51$), such mandates do not appear to be essential, as nine of the 38 countries with high NIHS coverage had no mandate.[16]

Access to effective screening

Mindful of the tracer indicator defined above, the *World Report on Hearing* calls for a 20% increase in effective NIHS coverage by 2030 as one of the targets for scaling up IPC-EHC services.[1] Specifically, countries with less than 50% coverage should aim for at least 50% coverage, countries with 50–80% coverage should aim for a 20% relative increase, countries with more than 80% coverage should aim for universal coverage, and countries with complete UNHS should aim for 95% or greater coverage.[1]

To further expand and improve NIHS programs around the world, the following initiatives could be considered.

- Countries with high NIHS coverage should ensure equitable access for their populations. They should volunteer to support countries with minimal NIHS programs.
- Governments should enact legislation to formalize the operation of NIHS programs. When possible, NIHS programs should be monitored through national committees on ear and hearing care.
- Data collection and tracking systems should be established, preferably from the beginning of NIHS program implementation, to track babies who have failed or missed screening and to provide systematic information on the coverage and quality of screening, intervention and rehabilitation services for individual children and their families, as well as on successes and gaps in these services. Ideally, these systems might use telemedicine components and bidirectional data flow between decentralized screening devices and hearing screening centers.[11]
- Creative and affordable solutions for making hearing technology more widely available need to be pursued.[25] This might include bulk purchases of hearing aids or implants.[12]

NIHS followed by early intervention has been shown to be effective, cost-efficient and an excellent investment of resources. The recent worldwide survey confirmed for the first time that NIHS benefits children, but also that global disparities remain.[26] As the world moves toward achieving the 2015 Sustainable Development Goals and universal health coverage, it is important that the needs of children with hearing loss are addressed and no one is left behind. To ensure all children achieve their 'highest attainable standard of health', the provision of NIHS as part of national plans for universal health coverage is a matter of equity and equality.

Key points – global status of newborn and infant hearing screening

- The effective coverage of NIHS services within a population is identified as a key indicator of global surveillance and monitoring of progress in ear and hearing care.
- A global survey has indicated that less than one-third of the world's population is covered by NIHS programs.
- Access to screening is linked to living standards, with the highest levels of screening coverage seen mostly in countries with the highest living standards.
- Many countries have high lost-to-follow-up rates, meaning that many children who fail initial hearing screening do not receive further intervention from diagnostic and treatment services.

References

1. World Health Organization. *World Report on Hearing.* Geneva: WHO, 2021. www.who.int/publications/i/item/world-report-on-hearing, last accessed 17 October 2021.
2. World Health Organization. *Childhood Hearing Loss: Strategies for Prevention and Care.* Geneva: WHO, 2016. www.who.int/docs/default-source/imported2/childhood-hearing-loss--strategies-for-prevention-and-care.pdf, last accessed 17 October 2021.

3. Yoshinaga-Itano C, Sedey AL, Coulter DK, Mehl AL. Language of early- and later-identified children with hearing loss. *Pediatrics* 1998;102:1161–71.
4. Yoshinaga-Itano C, Sedey AL, Wiggin M, Chung W. Early hearing detection and vocabulary of children with hearing loss. *Pediatrics* 2017;140:e20162964.
5. Neumann K, Gross M, Bottcher P et al. Effectiveness and efficiency of a universal newborn hearing screening in Germany. *Folia Phoniatr Logop* 2006;58:440–55.
6. Nelson HD, Bougatsos C, Nygren P; 2001 US Preventive Services Task Force. Universal newborn hearing screening: systematic review to update the 2001 US Preventive Services Task Force Recommendation. *Pediatrics* 2008;122:e266–76.
7. Pimperton H, Blythe H, Kreppner J et al. The impact of universal newborn hearing screening on long-term literacy outcomes: a prospective cohort study. *Arch Dis Child* 2016;101:9–15.
8. Ching TYC, Dillon H, Leigh G, Cupples L. Learning from the Longitudinal Outcomes of Children with Hearing Impairment (LOCHI) study: summary of 5-year findings and implications. *Int J Audiol* 2018;57(suppl 2):S105–11.
9. Wake M, Ching TY, Wirth K et al. Population outcomes of three approaches to detection of congenital hearing loss. *Pediatrics* 2016;137:e20151722.
10. Chiou ST, Lung HL, Chen LS et al. Economic evaluation of long-term impacts of universal newborn hearing screening. *Int J Audiol* 2017;56:46–52.
11. Sharma R, Gu Y, Ching TYC et al. Economic evaluations of childhood hearing loss screening programmes: a systematic review and critique. *Appl Health Econ Health Policy* 2019;17:331–57.
12. Wilson BS, Tucci DL, Merson MH, O'Donoghue GM. Global hearing health care: new findings and perspectives. *Lancet* 2017;390:2503–15.
13. World Health Organization. WHA48.9 Prevention of hearing impairment. Geneva: WHO, 1995. www.who.int/pbd/publications/wha_eb/wha48_9/en/, last accessed 17 October 2021.
14. World Health Organization. *Multi-Country Assessment of National Capacity to Provide Hearing Care.* Geneva: WHO, 2013. www.who.int/pbd/publications/WHOReportHearingCare_Englishweb.pdf, last accessed 17 October 2021.
15. World Health Organization. WHA70.13 Prevention of deafness and hearing loss. Geneva: WHO, 2017. http://apps.who.int/gb/ebwha/pdf_files/WHA70/A70_R13-en.pdf, last accessed 17 October 2021.

16. Neumann K, Euler HA, Chadha S, White KR. A survey on the global status of newborn and infant hearing screening. *J Early Hear Detect Interv* 2020;5:63–84.
17. Kral A. Auditory critical periods: a review from system's perspective. *Neuroscience* 2013;247:117–33.
18. World Health Organization. Newborn and infant hearing screening - Current issues and guiding principles for action. 2010. www.who.int/blindness/publications/Newborn_and_Infant_Hearing_Screening_Report.pdf, last accessed 17 October 2021.
19. Joint Committee on Infant Hearing. Year 2000 position statement: principles and guidelines for early hearing detection and intervention programs. *Am J Audiol* 2000;9:9–29.
20. Bussé AML, Hoeve HLJ, Nasserinejad K et al. Prevalence of permanent neonatal hearing impairment: systematic review and Bayesian meta-analysis. *Int J Audiology* 2020;59:475–85.
21. Ravi R, Gunjawate DR, Yerraguntla K et al. Follow-up in newborn hearing screening – a systematic review. *Int J Pediatr Otorhinolaryngol* 2016;90:29–36.
22. World Health Organization. *World Report on Disability*. Geneva: WHO, 2011. www.who.int/disabilities/world_report/2011/en/, last accessed 17 October 2021.
23. The Lancet. Hearing loss: time for sound action. *Lancet* 2017;390:2414.
24. World Health Organization. Deafness and hearing loss – key facts. Geneva: WHO, 2021. www.who.int/mediacentre/factsheets/fs300/en/, last accessed 17 October 2021.
25. Neumann K, Chadha S, Tavartkiladze G et al. Newborn and infant hearing screening facing globally growing numbers of people suffering from disabling hearing loss. *Int J Neonatal Screen* 2019;5:7.
26. Neumann K, Mathmann P, Chadha S et al. Newborn hearing screening benefits children, but global disparities persist. *J Clin Med* 2022;11:271.

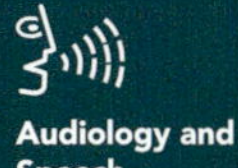

—

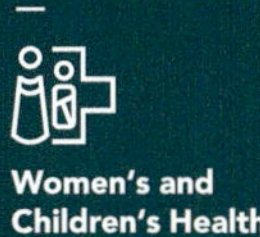

5 Genetic and CMV testing

Christine Yoshinaga-Itano

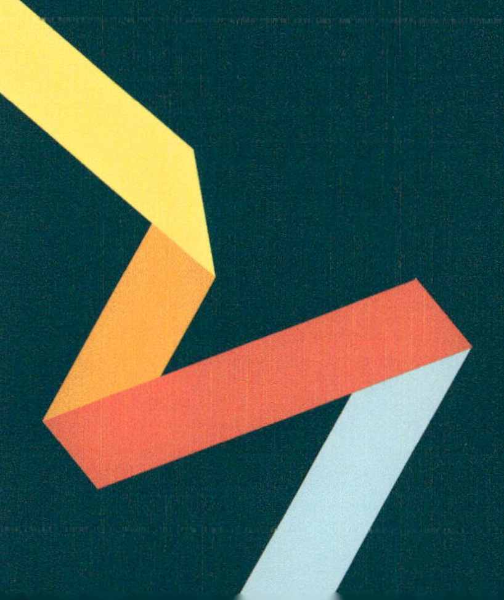

HEALTHCARE

Analysis of family history data from school-aged children in the USA has estimated that up to 60% of educationally significant congenital and early-onset hearing loss is caused by genetic factors.[1] Cytomegalovirus (CMV) infection causes hearing loss in up to an additional 20% of children (and 25% of all cases of pediatric hearing loss in the first 4 years of life).[2] Ideally, all families with children identified with hearing loss should be offered genetic and CMV screening to see if a cause can be determined, yet the majority of children with hearing loss do not undergo genetic testing, and few newborns are screened or tested for CMV in the immediate postnatal period.[1] It is wrongly believed by some that identifying the cause of hearing loss has no impact on the approach to treatment or that the timing of screening/testing does not matter. However, a definitive diagnosis of CMV must be reached shortly after birth to determine if the infection is congenital, while knowing that the hearing loss has a genetic etiology could alter a family's decision-making about interventions and could prevent serious medical complications in the future.

Genetic hearing loss

The majority of genetic hearing loss in the USA is inherited in an autosomal recessive pattern and often presents in the absence of a positive family history of hearing loss. Mutations in one gene, *GJB2*, which encodes the gap junction protein connexin 26, account for 50% of autosomal recessive early childhood hearing loss in many populations and 15–40% of all deaf individuals.[3,4]

Comprehensive genetic testing of a population of more than 1100 individuals with hearing loss, most of whom were younger than 17 years old, identified the underlying genetic cause of the hearing loss in 39%. The diagnostic rate rose to 48% among individuals with symmetrical hearing loss.[5]

A total of 49 genes were implicated in the etiology of the hearing loss, with variants of just four genes being identified most frequently:

- *GJB2* (22% of diagnoses overall)
- *STRC* (16%)
- *SLC26A4* (7%)
- *TECTA* (5%).

The study also identified variation in the causative genes depending on the extent of the hearing loss. For instance, mutations in *GJB2* were the most common cause of severe-to-profound hearing loss, accounting for 20% of diagnoses, but in mild-to-moderate hearing loss, variants of *STRC* accounted for 30% of diagnoses, with variants of *GJB2* accounting for 25% and variants of *TECTA* accounting for 7%.[5] Causative genes also varied with ethnicity.

Mutations in a second gap junction protein gene, *GJB6*, encoding connexin 30, have also been found in individuals with hearing loss. The impact of specific genes on the development of hearing loss is not yet known for most of the genes identified so far.

Hearing loss with a genetic etiology can be accompanied by other comorbidities; there are more than 400 genetic syndromes that include hearing loss as a feature, and more than 100 genes associated with non-syndromic genetic hearing loss.[6] Determining the cause of the hearing loss therefore informs the most effective approach to treatment.

Syndromic hearing loss accounts for an estimated 30% of genetic hearing loss cases. A few syndromes, such as Pendred (enlarged vestibular aqueduct, thyroid problems), Usher (retinitis pigmentosa), Waardenburg (pigmentary anomalies) and branchio-oto-renal (branchial arch and renal anomalies) syndromes, account for substantial percentages of hearing loss in some populations.[4,6–10]

Syndromic hearing loss may be transmitted as an autosomal recessive, autosomal dominant, X-linked or matrilineal trait. Reviews of individual conditions can be found in *Hereditary Hearing Loss and Its Syndromes* by Toriello and Smith (2013)[6] and the online database GeneReviews.[11]

Non-syndromic hearing loss accounts for an estimated 70% of genetic hearing loss cases. Non-syndromic hearing loss may be transmitted as an autosomal recessive (~80%), autosomal dominant (~15%), or X-linked trait (~1%).[4,6]

Matrilineal (mitochondrial) transmission of non-syndromic hearing loss occurs with a frequency of approximately 1% in Western nations but has a slightly higher incidence in Spain and East Asian countries, including China, Mongolia, Korea and Japan.[12,13]

Screening for genetic hearing loss

When screening cases of hearing loss for a possible genetic etiology, the American College of Medical Genetics and Genomics (ACMG) recommends that a comprehensive patient-focused medical and birth history is taken, together with a three-generation pedigree and family medical history and a physical examination (Figure 5.1).[4]

Patient medical and birth history can help in differentiating inherited causes of hearing loss from acquired hearing loss. It should cover:

- prenatal history – asking about maternal infections (such as CMV and rubella), illnesses (for example, syphilis), medication and drug exposures (including thalidomide and retinoic acid)[14,15]
- neonatal history – looking for factors such as premature birth, low birth weight, birth hypoxia, hyperbilirubinemia, sepsis and exposure to ototoxic medications
- postnatal history – including viral illnesses, bacterial meningitis, head trauma, noise exposure and exposure to ototoxic medications.

All children should have a comprehensive audiometric assessment of their hearing loss (as described in Chapter 10). Audiological characteristics such as degree, symmetry and type of hearing loss (sensorineural hearing loss [SNHL], conductive hearing loss [CHL] or mixed hearing loss) are significant for genetic etiology.

Pedigree and family medical history should include first- and second-degree relatives with hearing loss, or with features commonly associated with hearing loss (such as pigmentary, branchial or renal anomalies) or who experienced sudden cardiac death. The pattern of inheritance of the hearing loss should also be assessed: in individuals with a family history of dominant hearing loss, the cause was identified in 50% of cases in one study; the diagnostic rate fell to 41% in those with a family history of recessive hearing loss and to 37% in individuals with no family history of hearing loss.[5]

Other information that the ACMG guideline recommends be collected includes:

- ethnicity/country of origin
- common origin from ethnically/geographically isolated areas
- consanguinity.

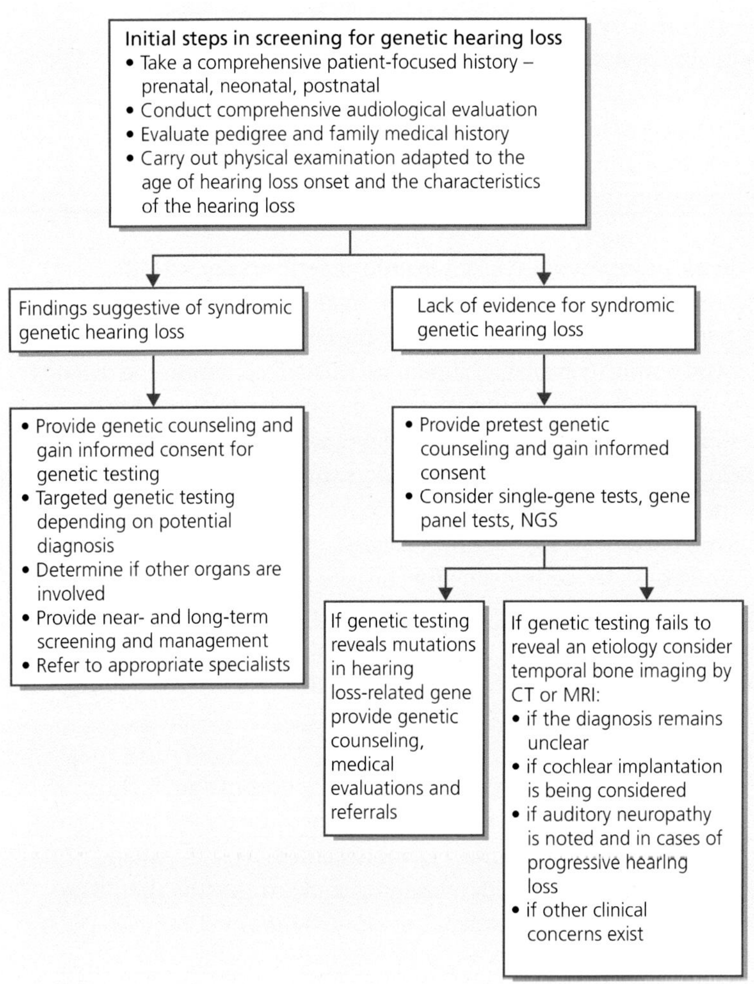

Figure 5.1 Decision-making hierarchy for the differentiation of syndromic and non-syndromic causes of hearing loss. NGS, next-generation sequencing. Adapted from www.acmg.net/PDFLibrary/Hearing-Loss-Clinical-Evaluation.pdf.

Physical examination should be customized based on the age of onset and the characteristics of the hearing loss. It should focus on dysmorphic and other physical findings including:[14,15]

- unusual facial appearance, with attention to asymmetry

- pigmentary anomalies
- neck, skin, facial or ear anomalies
- neurological abnormalities
- balance disturbances
- skeletal abnormalities
- other unusual physical findings.

When findings suggest a syndromic genetic etiology for the hearing loss, genetic counseling of individuals and/or their family is required. Then, with the patient's or the family's informed consent, genetic testing (if available) should be ordered to confirm the diagnosis. The cost of genetic screening can still be a barrier, but costs are decreasing. Testing is guided by the clinical findings, with the options available including single-gene tests, hearing loss sequencing panels, whole-exome sequencing (WES), whole-genome sequencing, chromosome analysis and microarray-based copy-number analysis.

The physician responsible for the care of the patient should arrange for any necessary testing to determine whether other organs are involved and, guided by the findings and associated manifestations of a suspected syndrome, provide near- and long-term screening and management and make appropriate referrals to specialists.

When physical findings suggestive of a syndrome are lacking and there is no suggestion of an environmental cause for the hearing loss, a tiered approach to diagnosis is implemented. As with patients with a syndromic genetic etiology, pretest genetic counseling should be provided and, with the patient's or family's informed consent, genetic testing can be requested. Currently, single-gene testing and testing to look for mutations in *GJB2* and *GJB6* may be employed initially, but as the costs of new sequencing technologies fall, it may eventually be more cost-effective to use next-generation sequencing (NGS) technologies as the initial test in the evaluation of hearing loss in these individuals.[4]

CMV testing should be done at the same time as genetic testing – and as soon as possible after birth – for infants with congenital hearing loss.

Failure to identify an underlying cause. Care for individuals with hearing loss for which genetic evaluation failed to identify an underlying cause should include periodic follow-up care every 3 years with a geneticist. Subtle features of syndromic forms of hearing loss may not be evident in the early years of life, but may manifest as an affected child grows toward adulthood. Also, as technology develops and medical knowledge advances, new genetic tests may become available, or the interpretation of previous test results may change. Periodic follow-up offers the opportunity to discuss developments or request additional testing and referral if required. The geneticist may also be able to identify clinical concerns unrelated to hearing loss and make appropriate referral for specialty care when appropriate.

All genetic test results – positive, negative and inconclusive – should be communicated through genetic counseling.

Cytomegalovirus testing and screening

CMV is the most common infectious cause of birth defects in the USA and about 6 out of 1000 babies are born with congenital CMV (cCMV) infection.[16–18] CMV infection is the leading non-genetic cause of hearing loss, affecting 10–20% of children with hearing loss in the USA.[2] A Dutch study reported that 8% of all SNHL was due to cCMV, but 23% of cases of profound hearing loss were due to cCMV.[19] About 25% of hearing loss reported in children by 4 years of age is caused by cCMV.[20]

Approximately 10–15% of infants with cCMV detected through universal screening are symptomatic at birth[21–24] and roughly 5% of infants with symptomatic cCMV (0.5% of all infected infants) will die. Of those infants who survive, 10–15% will have permanent sequelae, including permanent cognitive, hearing, visual and motor impairments, developmental delays and seizures.[2,17,18,23,25] Children with asymptomatic infection do not appear to be at significantly elevated risk for permanent cognitive[22,23] or visual disability,[26,27] but children with symptomatic or asymptomatic CMV have a high probability of delayed-onset or progressive hearing loss that can deteriorate from unilateral to bilateral or from mild or moderate to severe or profound. The prevalence of hearing loss in individuals with cCMV infection is around 13% (1 out of 3 symptomatic children and 1 out of 10 asymptomatic children).[17,21,28] Most SNHL in symptomatic children is bilateral whereas the majority of asymptomatic children have unilateral SNHL, at least initially.[17] Fluctuating hearing loss was present in 22.7% of children with hearing loss caused by CMV.[29]

In a study of children with hearing loss caused by cCMV, 50% experienced further deterioration of their hearing, with a median age at first progression of 18 months (range 2–70 months). Delayed-onset SNHL was observed in 18.2%, with the median age of detection being 27 months (range 25–62 months).[2] Fowler (2013)[2] states that approximately 33–50% of SNHL cases in cCMV-infected children have delayed onset.

Long-term audiological follow-up for at least 6 years is recommended in children with CMV infection if their hearing is assessed as being normal.[17]

Diagnosis. CMV can cross the placenta and infect a fetus when a pregnant woman is infected with CMV for the first time or is reinfected during pregnancy. The signs of cCMV infection that may be present at birth include:

- rash
- jaundice
- microcephaly
- intrauterine growth restriction (low birth weight)
- hepatosplenomegaly
- seizures
- retinitis.[30]

Fowler et al. (1992)[31] reported that, of the infants who were born with cCMV whose mothers had a primary infection during pregnancy, 15–33% developed SNHL. Of these, approximately 50% had bilateral hearing loss.[32,33]

cCMV infection can be diagnosed by testing a newborn baby's saliva, urine (preferred specimens) or blood, within 2–3 weeks after birth. The standard laboratory test for diagnosing cCMV infection is polymerase chain reaction (PCR) analysis of saliva (Figure 5.2), with urine usually collected and tested for confirmation. The reason for the confirmatory test on urine is that most CMV-seropositive mothers shed the virus in their breast milk, which can cause a false-positive result on saliva collected shortly after the baby has been breast-fed.

Currently, however, testing of newborns for CMV is not routinely performed, although targeted CMV testing of newborns who fail hearing screening occurs in some places. In the absence of screening, at least 50% of infants with symptomatic cCMV are not diagnosed or offered treatment.[19,34,35]

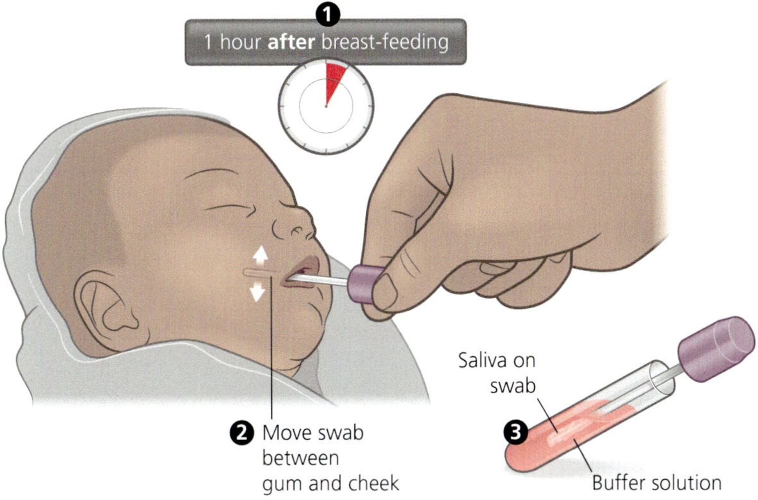

Figure 5.2 Technique for taking a saliva swab from a newborn for PCR diagnosis of cCMV infection.

Treatment. Because of safety concerns, antiviral treatment is typically restricted to children with symptomatic cCMV with additional CNS involvement.[18,36–40] Six weeks of antiviral treatment with intravenous ganciclovir has been demonstrated by one randomized controlled trial to be effective in reducing the progression of hearing loss in infants with symptomatic cCMV infections, with progression occurring in 21% of treated infants at 12 months versus 68% of untreated infants.[41]

However, a recently published long-term follow up of children with symptomatic cCMV who had received 6 weeks of ganciclovir treatment early in life found that they had the same severity of SNHL by 11–13 years of age as children who had not received ganciclovir treatment.[42,43] The severity of hearing loss was such that the children would be candidates for cochlear implantation.[42] The role of drug treatment in preventing progressive hearing loss therefore remains unclear.

Oral valganciclovir for 6 months has been reported in observational studies to reduce the frequency of hearing loss in children with symptomatic cCMV.[44] The major side effect is transient mild-to-moderate neutropenia.

Antiviral treatment may also be effective in preventing SNHL in children with asymptomatic cCMV; an observational study that monitored 18 children with asymptomatic cCMV for 4–10 years reported that SNHL occurred in 2 of 9 untreated children but 0 of 9 children treated with ganciclovir.[45] This finding requires confirmation in clinical trials. Antiviral treatment may also lead to improvement in hearing children with cCMV infection who develop late-onset SNHL;[46] this likewise requires confirmation. Concerns about toxicity, as well as limited data on long-term outcomes, have limited widespread use of these treatments.[47,48]

Even when families decide not to pursue antiviral treatment, knowing whether a child has had cCMV infection can alter the approach to rehabilitative treatment, monitoring of progression, amplification technology and early intervention services, because the needs of children with cCMV can differ from those of children with stable hearing loss.

Key points – genetic and CMV testing

- Up to 60% of educationally significant congenital and early-onset hearing loss has a genetic etiology.
- Most cases of genetic hearing loss are inherited in an autosomal recessive manner.
- There are more than 400 genetic syndromes that include hearing loss as a feature and an estimated 30% of cases of genetic hearing loss are syndromic.
- CMV is the leading non-genetic cause of hearing loss and 13% of infants with cCMV infection will have hearing loss.
- Infants with cCMV infections who are symptomatic at birth have an increased risk of permanent cognitive, hearing, visual and motor impairments, as well as developmental delays and seizures.
- Antiviral treatment has been investigated in children with cCMV but requires further evaluation; concern about toxicity and limited data on long-term outcomes have limited its widespread use.

References

1. Marazita ML, Ploughman LM, Rawlings B et al. Genetic epidemiological studies of early-onset deafness in the US school-age population. *Am J Med Genet* 1993;46:486–91.
2. Fowler KB. Congenital cytomegalovirus infection: audiologic outcome. *Clin Infect Dis* 2013;57(suppl 4):S182–4.
3. Pandya A, Arnos KS, Xia XJ et al. Frequency and distribution of GJB2 (connexin 26) and GJB6 (connexin 30) mutations in a large North American repository of deaf probands. *Genet Med* 2003;5:295–303.
4. Alford RL, Arnos KS, Fox M et al. American College of Medical Genetics and Genomics guideline for the clinical evaluation and etiologic diagnosis of hearing loss. *Genet Med* 2014;16:347–55.
5. Sloan-Heggen CM, Bierer AO, Shearer AE et al. Comprehensive genetic testing in the clinical evaluation of 1119 patients with hearing loss. *Hum Genet* 2016;135:441–50.
6. Toriello HV, Smith SD. *Hereditary Hearing Loss and Its Syndromes*, 3rd edn. New York: Oxford University Press, 2013.
7. Hereditary Hearing Loss Homepage. Syndromic hearing loss. https://hereditaryhearingloss.org/syndromic, last accessed 23 July 2021.
8. Kimberling WJ, Hildebrand MS, Shearer AE et al. Frequency of Usher syndrome in two pediatric populations: implications for genetic screening of deaf and hard of hearing children. *Genet Med* 2010;12:512–16.
9. Park HJ, Shaukat S, Liu XZ et al. Origins and frequencies of SLC26A4 (PDS) mutations in east and south Asians: global implications for the epidemiology of deafness. *J Med Genet* 2003;40:242–8.
10. Smith RJH. Branchiootorenal spectrum disorder. In: Adam MP, Ardinger HH, Pagon RA et al., eds. *GeneReviews* [Internet]. Seattle: University of Washington, 1999. www.ncbi.nlm.nih.gov/books/NBK1380/, last accessed 23 July 2021.
11. Adam MP, Ardinger HH, Pagon RA et al., eds. *GeneReviews* [Internet]. Seattle: University of Washington, 1993–2021. www.ncbi.nlm.nih.gov/books/NBK1116, last accessed 23 July 2021.
12. Li Z, Li R, Chen J et al. Mutational analysis of the mitochondrial 12S rRNA gene in Chinese pediatric subjects with aminoglycoside-induced and non-syndromic hearing loss. *Hum Genet* 2005;117:9–15.
13. Pandya A, Xia X, Radnaabazar J et al. Mutation in the mitochondrial 12S rRNA gene in two families from Mongolia with matrilineal aminoglycoside ototoxicity. *J Med Genet* 1997;34:169–72.

14. Dyer JJ, Strasnick B, Jacobson JT. Teratogenic hearing loss: a clinical perspective. *Am J Otol* 1998;19:671–8.
15. Takemori S, Tanaka Y, Suzuki JI. Thalidomide anomalies of the ear. *Arch Otolaryngol* 1976;102:425–7.
16. Kenneson A, Cannon MJ. Review and meta-analysis of the epidemiology of congenital cytomegalovirus (CMV) infection. *Rev Med Virol* 2007;17:253–76.
17. Goderis J, De Leenheer E, Smets K et al. Hearing loss and congenital CMV infection: a systematic review. *Pediatrics* 2014;134:972–82.
18. Swanson EC, Schleiss MR. Congenital cytomegalovirus infection: new prospects for prevention and therapy. *Pediatr Clin North Am* 2013;60:335–49.
19. Korver AM, de Vries JJ, Konings S et al. DECIBEL study: congenital cytomegalovirus infection in young children with permanent bilateral hearing impairment in the Netherlands. *J Clin Virol* 2009;46(suppl 4):S27–S31.
20. Morton CC, Nance WE. Newborn hearing screening – a silent revolution. *N Engl J Med* 2006;354:2151–64.
21. Dollard SC, Grosse SD, Ross DS. New estimates of the prevalence of neurological and sensory sequelae and mortality associated with congenital cytomegalovirus infection. *Rev Med Virol* 2007;17:355–63.
22. Cannon MJ, Griffiths PD, Aston V, Rawlinson WD. Universal newborn screening for congenital CMV infection: what is the evidence of potential benefit? *Rev Med Virol* 2014;24:291–307.
23. Cannon MJ, Grosse SD, Fowler KB. Cytomegalovirus epidemiology and public health impact. In: Reddehase MJ, ed. *Cytomegaloviruses: From Molecular Pathogenesis to Intervention,* volume II. Norfolk: Caister Academic Press, 2013:26–48.
24. Townsend CL, Forsgren M, Ahlfors K et al. Long-term outcomes of congenital cytomegalovirus infection in Sweden and the United Kingdom. *Clin Infect Dis* 2013;56:1232–9.
25. Grosse SD, Ross DS, Dollard SC. Congenital cytomegalovirus (CMV) infection as a cause of permanent bilateral hearing loss: a quantitative assessment. *J Clin Virol* 2008;41:57–62.
26. Anderson KS, Amos CS, Boppana S, Pass R. Ocular abnormalities in congenital cytomegalovirus infection. *J Am Optom Assoc* 1996;67:273–8.
27. Coats DK, Demmler GJ, Paysse EA et al. Ophthalmologic findings in children with congenital cytomegalovirus infection. *J AAPOS* 2000;4:110–16.
28. Dreher AM, Arora N, Fowler KB et al. Spectrum of disease and outcome in children with symptomatic congenital cytomegalovirus infection. *J Pediatr* 2014;164:855–9.

29. Fowler KB, McCollister FP, Dahle AJ et al. Progressive and fluctuating sensorineural hearing loss in children with asymptomatic congenital cytomegalovirus infection. *J Pediatr* 1997;130:624–30.
30. Centers for Disease Control and Prevention. *A Parent's Guide to Genetics & Hearing Loss*. www.cdc.gov/ncbddd/hearingloss/freematerials/parentsguide508.pdf, last accessed 23 July 2021.
31. Fowler KB, Stagno S, Pass RF et al. The outcome of congenital cytomegalovirus infection in relation to maternal antibody status. *N Engl J Med* 1992;326:663–7.
32. Foulon I, Naessens A, Foulon W et al. Hearing loss in children with a congenital cytomegalovirus infection related to the gestational age at which the maternal primary infection occurred. *Pediatrics* 2008;122:e1123–7.
33. Yamamoto AY, Mussi-Pinhata MM, Isaac M de L et al. Congenital cytomegalovirus infection as a cause of sensorineural hearing loss in a highly immune population. *Pediatr Infect Dis J* 2011;30:1043–6.
34. Avettand-Fenoël V, Marlin S, Vauloup-Fellous C et al. Congenital cytomegalovirus is the second most frequent cause of bilateral hearing loss in young French children. *J Pediatr* 2013;162:593–9.
35. Leung J, Cannon MJ, Grosse SD, Bialek SR. Laboratory testing and diagnostic coding for cytomegalovirus among privately insured infants in the United States: a retrospective study using administrative claims data. *BMC Pediatr* 2013;13:90.
36. Gandhi RS, Fernandez-Alvarez JR, Rabe H. Management of congenital cytomegalovirus infection: an evidence-based approach. *Acta Paediatr* 2010; 99:509–15.
37. Kadambari S, Williams EJ, Luck S et al. Evidence based management guidelines for the detection and treatment of congenital CMV. *Early Hum Dev* 2011;87:723–8.
38. Shin JJ, Keamy DG Jr, Steinberg EA. Medical and surgical interventions for hearing loss associated with congenital cytomegalovirus: a systematic review. *Otolaryngol Head Neck Surg* 2011;144:662–75.
39. Gwee A, Curtis N, Garland SM et al. Question 2: which infants with congenital cytomegalovirus infection benefit from antiviral therapy? *Arch Dis Child* 2014;99:597–601.
40. Marsico C, Kimberlin D. Congenital cytomegalovirus infection: advances and challenges in diagnosis, prevention and treatment. *Ital J Pediatr* 2017;43:38.

41. Kimberlin DW, Lin CY, Sanchez PJ et al. Effect of ganciclovir therapy on hearing in symptomatic congenital cytomegalovirus disease involving the central nervous system: a randomized, controlled trial. *J Pediatr* 2003;143:16–25.
42. Lanzieri TM, Caviness AC, Blum P et al. Progressive, long-term hearing loss in congenital CMV disease after ganciclovir therapy. *J Pediatric Infect Dis Soc* 2022;11:16–23.
43. Schleiss MR. Antiviral therapy and its long-term impact on hearing loss caused by congenital cytomegalovirus: much remains to be learned! *J Pediatric Infect Dis Soc* 2022; in press.
44. del Rosal T, Baquero-Artigao F, Blázquez D et al. Treatment of symptomatic congenital cytomegalovirus infection beyond the neonatal period. *J Clin Virol* 2012;55:72–4.
45. Lackner A, Acham A, Alborno T et al. Effect on hearing of ganciclovir therapy for asymptomatic congenital cytomegalovirus infection: four to 10 year follow up. *J Laryngol Otol* 2009;123:391–6.
46. Amir J, Attias J, Pardo J. Treatment of late-onset hearing loss in infants with congenital cytomegalovirus infection. *Clin Pediatr (Phila)* 2014;53:444–8.
47. Plosa EJ, Esbenshade JC, Fuller MP, Weitkamp JH. Cytomegalovirus infection. *Pediatr Rev* 2012;33:156–63.
48. Hamilton ST, van Zuylen W, Shand A et al. Prevention of congenital cytomegalovirus complications by maternal and neonatal treatments: a systematic review. *Rev Med Virol* 2014;24:420–33.

Further reading and resources

Genetic testing

Center for Mitochondrial & Epigenomic Medicine, Children's Hospital of Philadelphia. MITOMAP (human mitochondrial genome database). www.mitomap.org/MITOMAP

Centers for Disease Control and Prevention. *A Parent's Guide to Genetics and Hearing Loss*. www.cdc.gov/ncbddd/hearingloss/freematerials/parentsguide508.pdf

Deafness Variation Database. https://deafnessvariationdatabase.org

Harvard Medical School Center for Hereditary Deafness. *Understanding the Genetics of Deafness. A Guide for Patients and Families*. https://projects.iq.harvard.edu/files/centerforhereditarydeafness/files/understanding_the_genetics_of_deafness.pdf

Hereditary Hearing Loss Homepage. https://hereditaryhearingloss.org/ (provides an up-to-date overview of the genetics of hereditary hearing loss)

National Institute on Deafness and Other Communication Disorders. Hearing, ear infections, and deafness. www.nidcd.nih.gov/health/hearing/

Shared Harvard Inner-Ear Laboratory Database (SHIELD). https://shield.hms.harvard.edu/index.html

University of Iowa, AudioGene. https://audiogene.eng.uiowa.edu

University of Maryland gene Expression Analysis Resource (gEAR). https://umgear.org

US National Library of Medicine, MedlinePlus. Nonsyndromic hearing loss. https://medlineplus.gov/genetics/condition/nonsyndromic-hearing-loss/

CMV testing

Centers for Disease Control and Prevention. Babies born with congenital cytomegalovirus. www.cdc.gov/cmv/congenital-infection.html

East of England Neonatal ODN, National Health Service. Congenital cytomegalovirus guideline. www.eoeneonatalpccsicnetwork.nhs.uk/neonatal/downloads/congenital-cytomegalovirus-guideline

Griffiths PG, Heath P, Hollins Martin C et al. We need to talk about CMV. CMV Action, 2015. https://cmvaction.org.uk/resources/publications

National CMV Foundation. www.nationalcmv.org/about-us/advocacy

UpToDate. Congenital cytomegalovirus infection: clinical features and diagnosis. www.uptodate.com/contents/congenital-cytomegalovirus-infection-clinical-features-and-diagnosis

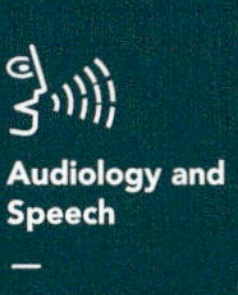

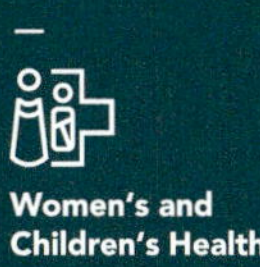

6 Medical evaluation and management of permanent childhood hearing loss

Tony KS Sirimanna and Waheeda Pagarkar

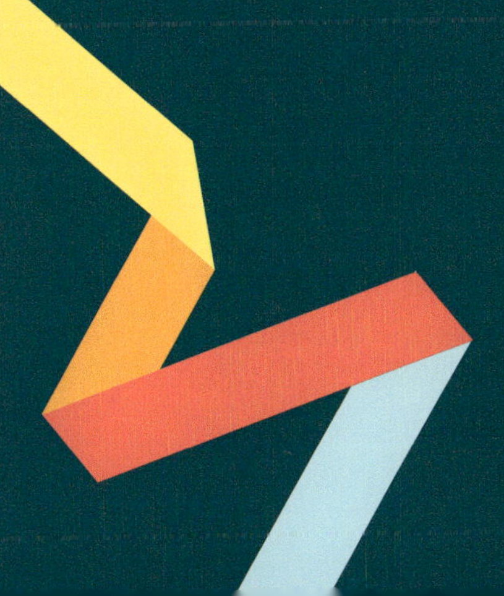

HEALTHCARE

Medical evaluation of children with PHL should be initiated alongside audiological evaluation and early intervention programs to investigate the cause of the PHL and consider associated medical comorbidities that may influence the management of the children and the counseling of their families. In one study, 41% of children with PHL were found to have associated disabilities that might require additional resources for management.[1] Hearing loss may also be the first noticeable manifestation of a systemic illness such as cCMV infection or neurometabolic conditions.

Medical evaluation will often lead to referral to other specialties, and suggestions of medical or surgical treatments. This should be considered early, as any delay may have a lasting impact on the outcome.

Medical etiologies of hearing loss

The etiology of PHL is changing as a result of more widespread use of immunizations (mumps, measles, rubella, meningitis, etc.) and better pre-, peri- and postnatal care. The commonest cause of bilateral PHL in children is genetic (see Chapter 5), while unilateral loss is most often caused by abnormalities of the temporal bone (Table 6.1).[2]

Specific genes may be identified only in approximately two-thirds of those suspected to have genetic hearing loss,[2] but with the advent of 'deafness panels' and WES, this is expected to rise in the future.[3] In spite of robust investigatory protocols, at best only 60–65% of children with PHL have an etiologic diagnosis. This could be due to conditions yet to be recognized (for example, associated with new genes) or gaps in investigation protocols.

Although newborn hearing screens can detect most children with PHL, some children will develop hearing loss later in life (postnatal onset or progressive hearing loss), and will be missed by the newborn screen. Likewise, hearing loss that is mild or involves a single frequency may be missed. Children with auditory neuropathy may not be detected by hearing screens that use only OAE. For this reason, surveillance of hearing is important, and the JCIH has recommended continued monitoring of children with a high risk of hearing loss (Table 6.2).[4]

TABLE 6.1

Etiology of permanent hearing loss in infants and children

Etiology	Details/examples
Genetic hearing loss*	• Causes 50% or more cases of PHL
Syndromic	• Responsible for 30% of genetic cases of PHL, >300 syndromes described; e.g. Pendred, Waardenburg, Usher, branchio-oto-renal, Alport, Alström, Norrie and craniofacial syndromes such as Down and Apert
Non-syndromic	• Responsible for 70% of genetic cases; approximately 120 genes have been identified
Autosomal recessive	• Responsible for 80% of non-syndromic cases • Connexin 26 is the commonest genetic etiology, causing 50% of recessive cases
Autosomal dominant	• *KCNQ4, TECTA*
X-linked	• *POU3F4*
Mitochondrial	• m.1555A>G
Antenatal and perinatal factors	
Intrauterine insults	• Infections: CMV, rubella, toxoplasma, syphilis, herpes, Zika, HIV • Teratogens: fetal alcohol syndrome, phenytoin • Maternal diabetes
Birth-related insults	• Birth asphyxia • Intracranial hemorrhage
Postnatal	• Severe neonatal jaundice • Prolonged ventilation and ECMO • Sepsis and meningitis
Temporal bone malformations	• Cochlear nerve hypoplasia • Cochlea hypoplasia • Enlarged vestibular aqueducts • Incomplete partitioning malformations

CONTINUED

TABLE 6.1 CONTINUED

Etiology of permanent hearing loss in infants and children

Etiology	Details/examples
Craniofacial malformations	• Microtia • Cleft palate • Craniosynostosis syndromes
Infections	• Bacterial meningitis • Infectious labyrinthitis • Lyme disease • Measles, mumps, varicella • Tuberculosis
Traumatic	• Temporal bone fracture • Barotrauma • Noise-induced • Perilymphatic fistula
Ototoxic medications	• Aminoglycosides • Cisplatin • Loop diuretics
Tumors	• Vestibular schwannoma, • Neurofibromatosis type 2 • Astrocytoma • Medulloblastoma
Autoimmune conditions	• Cogan syndrome • Systemic lupus erythematosus • Juvenile idiopathic arthritis (formerly juvenile rheumatoid arthritis) • Wegener granulomatosis • Sjögren syndrome • Behçet disease • Antiphospholipid syndrome • Anticardiolipin syndrome • Hashimoto thyroiditis

CONTINUED

TABLE 6.1 CONTINUED

Etiology of permanent hearing loss in infants and children

Etiology	Details/examples
Systemic/vascular conditions	• Diabetes mellitus • Sickle cell disease • Hypothyroidism
Neurodegenerative conditions	• Mitochondrial (MELAS) • Mucopolysaccharidosis
Unknown etiology	• Meniere's disease • Otosclerosis

*Different mutations in the same gene can be associated with different types of hearing loss; some genes are associated with both syndromic and non-syndromic forms of genetic hearing loss.
ECMO, extracorporeal membrane oxygenation; MELAS, mitochondrial encephalopathy, lactic acidosis and stroke-like episodes.

TABLE 6.2

Risk factors for early childhood hearing loss in infants who pass newborn screening[4]

Perinatal factors

- Family history of permanent childhood hearing loss
- Neonatal intensive care for more than 5 days
- Hyperbilirubinemia with exchange transfusion
- Aminoglycoside administration for more than 5 days
- Asphyxia or hypoxic ischemic encephalopathy
- ECMO
- In utero infections: toxoplasma, rubella, herpes, syphilis, CMV, Zika
- Craniofacial malformations, including cleft palate, microcephaly, hydrocephalus, microtia, microphthalmia, temporal bone anomaly
- Syndromes associated with hearing loss

CONTINUED

TABLE 6.2 CONTINUED

Risk factors for early childhood hearing loss in infants who pass newborn screening[4]

Perinatal or postnatal factors

- Culture-positive infections associated with hearing loss, including confirmed bacterial or viral meningitis (especially herpes, varicella) and encephalitis
- Events associated with hearing loss, including trauma to basal skull and temporal bone, and chemotherapy
- Caregiver concern regarding hearing, language, developmental delay, developmental regression

ECMO, extracorporeal membrane oxygenation.

Medical evaluation

Depending on local resources, medical evaluation of a child with PHL may be performed by a range of professionals, including audiovestibular and ear, nose and throat physicians, pediatricians and geneticists. Regardless of who performs the evaluation, the medical professional should be sensitive to the priorities, preferences and emotions of the family when arranging medical evaluations, and should work with the audiology and wider multidisciplinary team caring for the child to ensure seamless care.

The role of the medical professional is to perform a full diagnostic evaluation of the infant/child, including arranging investigations. They may also be the primary medical care provider, and have responsibility for monitoring the overall development and wellbeing of the child, and addressing family concerns as they occur.

History. The clinical history should include a detailed antenatal, birth and postnatal history, developmental milestones, systemic symptoms and family history, including parental consanguinity. If the cause of hearing loss is not apparent, any history of individual etiologies of hearing loss, such as meningitis, should be looked into.

Clinical examination should include detailed top-to-toe general and systemic examination, looking for features of syndromes and pointers to the etiology of hearing loss, including:

- ear/neck pits and tags
- spinal abnormalities
- facial dysmorphism
- thyroid swelling
- nail hypoplasia
- cleft palate (including submucous cleft)
- cardiac murmur
- pigmentary abnormalities.

All children should have a detailed examination of the eyes and a clinical evaluation of the vestibular system. The latter can be done by an age-appropriate assessment of balance, head thrust test and appropriate neonatal reflexes (for example, Farmer's rotation test, Moro reflex, labyrinthine righting reflex). Vestibular function assessment is discussed in more detail on page 73.

Investigations

Several guidelines have been written for etiologic investigations of hearing loss in children with PHL, and particular investigations depend on the degree and type of hearing loss (sensorineural/conductive/auditory neuropathy) and whether it is unilateral or bilateral.[5] Etiologic investigation is an ongoing process, and children who have not had an etiologic diagnosis should be periodically re-evaluated, as some symptoms could appear with the passage of time (for instance, visual loss in Usher syndrome).

CMV DNA detection is conducted on a saliva swab or urine sample if the child is younger than 1 year. A positive result in a child less than 3 weeks old is diagnostic of cCMV infection. After 3 weeks of age, a positive result could be due to postnatally acquired CMV and therefore testing for CMV DNA on the neonatal blood spot is required to confirm diagnosis.

In children older than 1 year, serological testing can be performed to look for immunoglobulin G (IgG) antibodies against CMV.

A negative result excludes cCMV but, if testing is positive, a CMV PCR test on the neonatal blood spot is needed to confirm diagnosis.

The sensitivity of detection of CMV DNA on the neonatal blood spot is close to 80%, and a negative result does not exclude a diagnosis of cCMV. cCMV can be ruled out in infants if testing for maternal IgG antibodies to CMV is negative.

As discussed in Chapter 5, cCMV is the cause of hearing loss in 10–20% of children with SNHL. CMV testing is a priority investigation in babies born with SNHL, as a diagnosis of cCMV would merit consideration of antiviral treatment (see page 55). This is thought to limit the progressive decline in hearing that can occur with cCMV infection and improve neurodevelopmental outcome.[6]

The prevalence of hearing loss in children with cCMV infection is around 13% (1 out of 3 symptomatic children and 1 out of 10 asymptomatic children). The hearing loss is often severe to profound. Long-term audiological follow-up for at least 6 years is recommended if hearing is normal.[7]

Inner ear imaging. MRI of the inner ears is indicated in SNHL and mixed hearing loss. Common abnormalities detected include enlarged vestibular aqueducts, hypoplastic cochlear nerves and incomplete partitioning of the cochlea (Figure 6.1). MRI findings may prompt genetic investigations. Imaging should include the brain to look for evidence of cCMV and the basal ganglia in infants with kernicterus.

MRI is a safe investigation, but requires the infant to stay still for the duration of the scan; therefore, it is best performed in the first 12 weeks of life, with a view to avoiding sedation.

A CT scan of the petrous bones is indicated in children with permanent CHL. A CT scan, as well as MRI, can be used in cases of bacterial meningitis to look for labyrinthitis ossificans. CT scans are best avoided in infancy because of the exposure to radiation. However, if needed, cone beam CT helps to focus on the area of interest and limit radiation exposure. Radiological investigation is the highest-yielding test for children with bilateral as well as unilateral SNHL.[8–10]

Genetic testing has evolved in recent years, particularly with the advent of NGS and the creation of a 'deafness panel', in which several

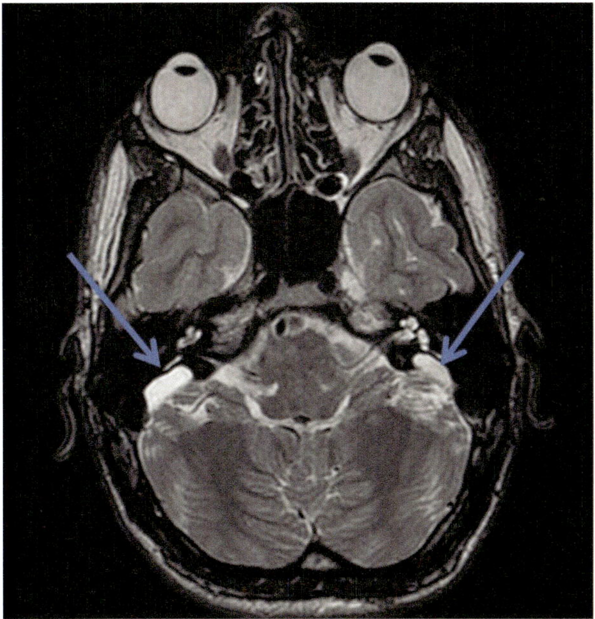

Figure 6.1 Axial MRI scan of the internal auditory meatuses showing enlarged endolymphatic sacs (arrows).

genetic mutations associated with syndromic and non-syndromic hearing loss can be tested together, and the availability of WES. This has greatly increased the yield of genetic testing.[11]

Where the panel test is not available, further genetic testing will be guided by clinical features, for instance, testing for Pendred syndrome in children with bilaterally enlarged vestibular aqueducts or for branchio-oto-renal syndrome if preauricular pits are present. Other specific genetic tests are indicated in Table 6.3.

In all cases, parents should be provided with verbal and written information on genetic investigations and informed consent should be obtained.

Ophthalmic evaluation. Concomitant ophthalmic pathologies have been found in 21–48% of children diagnosed with congenital SNHL, of which the most common were refractive pathologies.[12,13] These are likely to further compromise sensory input to hearing-impaired children and merit consideration during management. Ophthalmic

TABLE 6.3

Specific genetic tests in children with hearing loss

- Connexin 26 is the commonest genetic cause of SNHL and testing should be requested for all children with bilateral SNHL
- Mitochondrial mutations in m.1555A>G cause susceptibility to aminoglycoside toxicity. This test is requested for children exposed to aminoglycosides, those with a history of hearing loss on the maternal side of the family and those with high-frequency SNHL
- Chromosomal studies and microarray testing are requested for children with dysmorphic features and developmental delay
- For children with ANSD, specific genetic tests look for mutations in the otoferlin (normally associated with bilateral severe-to-profound hearing loss), pejvakin and *MPZ* (myelin protein zero) genes

evaluation is recommended in all children with permanent hearing impairment.[14]

Common conditions with eye involvement in children with hearing loss include syndromes such as Usher, CHARGE (coloboma, heart defects, atresia choanae, growth retardation, genital abnormalities and ear abnormalities), Stickler, Alport, Alström, DIDMOAD (diabetes insipidus, diabetes mellitus, optic atrophy and deafness), TORCH (toxoplasmosis, other agents, rubella, CMV and herpes simplex) and Norrie disease, and cerebral palsy.

Children should be referred for electrophysiological studies (electroretinography) if they have a history of delayed motor milestones, symptoms suggestive of Usher syndrome or optic atrophy.

Family audiograms. Although not backed by a high level of evidence, family audiograms may often uncover undetected hearing loss among siblings and parents. They may be useful in the interpretation of genetic test results.

Electrocardiograms are indicated in children with profound SNHL and delayed motor milestones to look for prolonged QT syndrome (Jervell and Lange-Nielsen syndrome). Although very rare, this is an important diagnosis to make as treatment significantly reduces mortality.[15]

Serology for congenital infections such as toxoplasma, rubella, syphilis, Zika virus and HIV may be indicated depending on clinical suspicion. Test results in a neonate should be interpreted in the context of maternal serology, and the opinion of a specialist in infectious disease may be required.

Kidney ultrasound scans are indicated if there is a family history of renal disease, clinical suspicion of syndromes with kidney involvement (such as branchio-oto-renal syndrome), permanent CHL or enlarged vestibular aqueducts.

Metabolic screens on blood and urine are performed in cases with a history of developmental delay and visual difficulty.

Investigation of potential autoimmune disease, including testing for antinuclear antibodies and an autoimmune screen, is indicated in cases with systemic symptoms such as fever, skin rash or joint swelling.

Vestibular function assessment. Clinical evaluation of the vestibular system should be done in all children with PHL. Where facilities are available, vestibular function tests may be requested for children who have:

- delayed motor milestones
- vestibular malformations
- syndromes with known vestibular involvement (for example, Usher syndrome)
- vertigo/dizziness
- progressive hearing loss.

Vestibular function assessment should also be performed before cochlear implantation.

Other investigations. Specific investigations should be guided by clinical features. For instance, urine dipstick testing is used to look for hematuria in Alport syndrome, while thyroid function tests are indicated in adolescents with confirmed Pendred syndrome.

Medical considerations when managing hearing loss

Glue ear can delay the diagnosis of underlying PHL and can increase its severity, causing difficulties in effective amplification. In children with SNHL and glue ear, the decision to place ventilation tubes should be considered carefully, for example, in cases when the degree of hearing loss is unlikely to be managed by amplification alone, and in children undergoing cochlear implant assessment. For children with underlying craniofacial anomalies such as cleft palate and Down syndrome, with a high risk of longstanding middle ear dysfunction, bilateral glue ear is best managed by amplification devices initially. Surgical intervention can be considered when amplification is not an option, is limited by compliance or is not effective, or when indicated due to unsafe middle ear pathology. Parents should be counseled about potential side effects, such as ear discharge, which can affect regular hearing aid use.

Vestibular hypofunction occurs in 30–70% of children with SNHL, depending on the degree of hearing loss and the tests done to assess vestibular function. This can vary from mild dysfunction to bilateral vestibular loss, and often correlates with the severity of hearing loss. It can impact on the motor development of the child and cause balance difficulties. Age of independent walking is delayed beyond 18 months and children will often require physiotherapy support.[16] Parents of children with vestibular hypofunction must be counseled about the risk of drowning during underwater swimming.

Recognition of vestibular hypofunction is also important as it draws attention to particular etiologies of hearing loss, including cochlear vestibular abnormalities, cCMV infection, Usher syndrome, and Jervell and Lange-Nielsen syndrome. In children with SNHL and vestibular hypofunction, investigations should include CMV testing and MRI. If these tests do not indicate the etiology, detailed genetic testing should follow.

Medical treatment and monitoring is an option in some circumstances, including for intrauterine infections such as cCMV, toxoplasma and syphilis. The control of underlying medical conditions such as sickle cell anemia is likely to limit the hearing loss caused, while the investigation of hearing loss may uncover neurodegenerative conditions such as mucopolysaccharidosis, for which early treatment is crucial to a better prognosis.

Sudden SNHL may be managed with steroid medication. Children with long QT syndrome may need a beta-blocker or a pacemaker, and should be counseled to avoid certain medications that may precipitate a cardiac arrest. Individuals with the mitochondrial m.1555A>G mutation should be advised to avoid aminoglycosides and counseled about the possibility of loss of hearing with their continued use. Children with enlarged vestibular aqueducts will need advice regarding avoidance of large pressure changes and head injuries to reduce the risk of a decline in their hearing. These children should be evaluated for Pendred syndrome.

Thyroid function monitoring from the onset of adolescence is necessary in individuals with Pendred syndrome. Treatment of congenital hypothyroidism may limit hearing loss.

Children with bacterial meningitis showing changes of labyrinthitis ossificans on CT/MRI merit urgent consideration for cochlear implantation.

In rare instances, intracranial tumors can present as hearing loss and may be treatable.

Auditory neuropathy. Medical input in the management of auditory neuropathy is important for various reasons.

- The auditory neuropathy may be a manifestation of a generalized neurological condition, such as Fredriech's ataxia or leukodystrophies, or there could be an opportunity to treat the condition (for example, Brown-Vialetto-Van Laere syndrome);[17] a neurological referral is often indicated.
- Up to 50% of babies with an auditory neuropathy-like picture will spontaneously improve in the first year of life (particularly preterm babies with a stormy perinatal course).
- Decisions for cochlear implantation may often be delayed due to the variable prognosis in children with auditory neuropathy.

Psychological comorbidities. Emotional and behavioral difficulties are twice as common in children with hearing loss as in those without, and there is a strong association between hearing loss and internalizing behaviors (depression, anxiety) in children.[18,19] Conduct and hyperactivity disorders, as well as emotional and executive function problems, among children with PHL may be related to poor language development. These problems are more prevalent in children with additional disabilities.

Psychological disorders may be difficult to diagnose and assess in children with PHL due to language difficulties, and behavior difficulties may persist despite early management of hearing loss.

Progressive and sudden hearing loss. Children with PHL need ongoing monitoring as 30–50% may show further progression of their hearing loss. Medical investigation may identify children at risk of progressive hearing loss, for instance those with enlarged vestibular aqueducts, m.1555A>G mutations or cCMV.

The parents of children receiving ototoxic medication for the treatment of other conditions (such as aminoglycosides for cystic fibrosis or *cis*-platinum for malignancies) should be counseled about the risk of progressive hearing loss. The use of such medications has been subject to potential litigation claims.[20]

There is some evidence to support intratympanic and oral steroids for the management of sudden hearing loss.[21]

Auditory implants. Medical conditions will influence decision-making around cochlear implants. Children with meningitis should be fast tracked for implants while those with absent cochlear nerves will not be candidates for this surgery. Progressive neurodegenerative conditions heavily influence the decision to offer implants. All children receiving cochlear implants should be offered meningitis vaccination.

X-linked deafness may be associated with an intraoperative cerebrospinal fluid leakage (CSF gusher) during implant surgery and adequate precautions must be taken.

Children with microtia can be offered both bone-anchored hearing aids (BAHA) and ear plastic surgery. Children with chronically discharging ears can be considered for BAHA.

Middle ear implants can be considered for suitable candidates.

Genetic counseling

The families of children with genetic hearing loss will require counseling about the potential of hearing loss in future offspring. This may affect planning for further pregnancies, including consideration of preimplantation genetic diagnosis, amniocentesis or in vitro fertilization using a donor.

Children with hearing loss will need appropriate genetic counseling when they reach adulthood and begin to consider starting their own families.

A further consideration is that a positive genetic test result (such as for the mitochondrial mutation m.1555A>G) may have implications for the extended family.

Gene therapy for hearing loss

With progress in genomic medicine, attempts have been made to treat mouse models of human deafness with gene therapy with variable success. Issues to be considered are the timing of therapy, its mode of delivery, viral vectors and stem cells. Although much more work is required, there is optimism that such research will be extended to people in the decades to come.[22]

Key points – medical evaluation and management of permanent hearing loss

- Medical evaluation can help determine the cause and guide the management of PHL in children.
- Bilateral PHL most commonly has a genetic cause; unilateral PHL is most commonly the result of abnormalities of the temporal bone.
- The degree and type of hearing loss, and whether it is bilateral or unilateral, influence the specific etiologic investigations undertaken.
- CMV is a priority investigation in babies born with SNHL because a positive diagnosis merits consideration of antiviral treatment.
- Medical input into the management of a range of conditions associated with hearing loss, such as glue ear, vestibular hypofunction and auditory neuropathy, can ensure that optimal approaches are employed.

References

1. Tufatulin GS, Koroleva IV, Artyushkin SA, Yanov YK. Kompleksnye narusheniya u detei s sensonevral'noi tugoukhost'yu – vliyanie na diagnostiku patologii slukha i slukhoprotezirovanie [Complex disorders in children with sensorineural hearing loss – influence on the diagnosis of hearing pathology and hearing aid]. *Vestn Otorinolaringol* 2020;85:30–34.
2. van Beeck Calkoen EA, Engel MSD, van de Kamp JM et al. The etiological evaluation of sensorineural hearing loss in children. *Eur J Pediatr* 2019;178:1195–205.
3. Božanić Urbančič N, Battelino S, Tesovnik T, Trebušak Podkrajšek K. The importance of early genetic diagnostics of hearing loss in children. *Medicina (Kaunas)* 2020;56:471.
4. Joint Committee on Infant Hearing. Year 2019 position statement: principles and guidelines for early hearing detection and intervention programs. *J Early Hear Detect Interv* 2019;4:1–44.
5. British Association of Audiovestibular Physicians. Documents, guidelines and clinical standards. www.baap.org.uk/documents-guidelines-pathways-and-clinical-standards.html, last accessed 3 June 2021.
6. Marsico C, Kimberlin DW. Congenital cytomegalovirus infection: advances and challenges in diagnosis, prevention and treatment. *Ital J Pediatr* 2017;43:38.
7. Goderis J, De Leenheer E, Smets K et al. Hearing loss and congenital CMV infection: a systematic review. *Pediatrics* 2014;134:972–82.
8. Kachniarz B, Chen JX, Gilani S, Shin JJ. Diagnostic yield of MRI for pediatric hearing loss: a systematic review. *Otolaryngol Head Neck Surg* 2015;152:5–22.
9. van Beeck Calkoen EA, Merkus P, Goverts ST et al. Evaluation of the outcome of CT and MR imaging in pediatric patients with bilateral sensorineural hearing loss. *Int J Pediatr Otorhinolaryngol* 2018; 108:180–5.
10. Ropers FG, Dekkers OM, Rotteveel LJC. Imaging for pediatric unilateral sensorineural hearing loss – reply. *JAMA Otolaryngol Head Neck Surg* 2019;145:1083.
11. Sloan-Heggen CM, Bierer AO, Shearer AE et al. Comprehensive genetic testing in the clinical evaluation of 1119 patients with hearing loss. *Hum Genet* 2016;135:441–50.
12. Gruber M, Brown C, Mahadevan M, Neeff M. Hearing loss and ophthalmic pathology in children diagnosed before and after the implementation of a universal hearing screening program. *Isr Med Assoc J* 2019;21:607–11.

13. Batson S, Kelly K, Morrison D, Virgin F. Ophthalmologic abnormalities in children with congenital sensorineural hearing loss. *J Binocul Vis Ocul Motil* 2019;69:126–30.
14. NDCS/SENSE. Vision care for deaf children and young people. Guidelines for professionals. www.ndcs.org.uk/media/4141/qs_vision_care_for_deaf_children_and_young_people_2009.pdf, last accessed 4 November 2021.
15. Schwartz PJ, Periti M, Malliani A. The long Q-T syndrome. *Am Heart J* 1975;89:378–90.
16. Janky KL, Thomas MLA, High RR et al. Predictive factors for vestibular loss in children with hearing loss. *Am J Audiol* 2018;27:137–46.
17. Menezes MP, O'Brien K, Hill M et al. Auditory neuropathy in Brown-Vialetto-Van Laere syndrome due to riboflavin transporter RFVT2 deficiency. *Dev Med Child Neurol* 2016; 58:848–54.
18. Bigler D, Burke K, Laureano N et al. Assessment and treatment of behavioral disorders in children with hearing loss: a systematic review. *Otolaryngol Head Neck Surg* 2019;160:36–48.
19. Stevenson J, Kreppner J, Pimperton H et al. Emotional and behavioural difficulties in children and adolescents with hearing impairment: a systematic review and meta-analysis. *Eur Child Adolesc Psychiatry* 2015;24:477–96.
20. van As JW, van den Berg H, van Dalen EC. Platinum-induced hearing loss after treatment for childhood cancer. *Cochrane Database Syst Rev* 2016;2016:CD010181.
21. Reading JCS, Hall A, Nash R. Paediatric sudden sensorineural hearing loss: pooled analysis and systematic review. *J Int Adv Otol* 2021;17:64–71.
22. Omichi R, Shibata SB, Morton CC, Smith RJH. Gene therapy for hearing loss. *Hum Mol Genet* 2019;28:R65–79.

Further reading and resources

American Academy of Pediatrics Task Force for Improving Newborn Hearing Screening, Diagnosis and Intervention. Early hearing detection and intervention (EHDI) guidelies for pediatric medical home providers. 2010. https://health.utah.gov/cshcn/pdf/EHDI/EHDI%20Guidelines%20for%20Pediatricians.pdf, last accessed 9 June 2022.

Liming BJ, Carter J, Cheng A et al. International Pediatric Otolaryngology Group (IPOG) consensus recommendations: hearing loss in the pediatric patient. *Int J Pediatr Otorhinolaryngol* 2016;90:251–8.

Sung V, Downie L, Paxton GA et al. Childhood Hearing Australasian Medical Professionals network: consensus guidelines on investigation and clinical management of childhood hearing loss. *J Paediatr Child Health* 2019;55:1013–22.

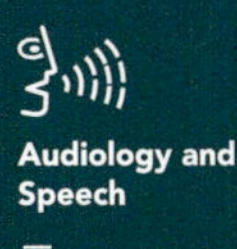

—

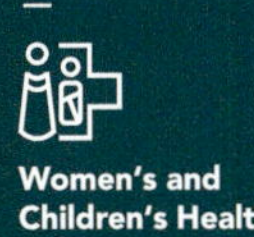

7 Middle ear effusion and other barriers to timely diagnosis

Lisa L Hunter

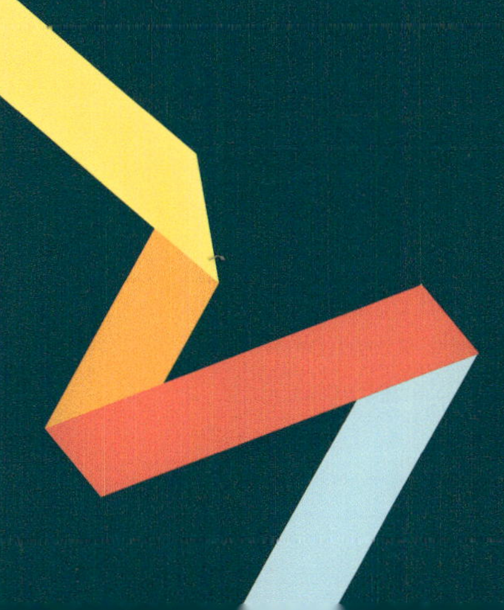

HEALTHCARE

The first year after a baby's birth presents a steep learning curve for the baby and its parents. Human communication, both verbal and non-verbal, normally unfolds like a well-synchronized dance between infant and parents. This interaction lays the foundation for language that is essential to social skills, reading and later academic development. For infants with PHL, any delay in access to auditory stimulation can result in long-term developmental consequences.[1,2] The EHDI 1–3–6 (preferably 1–2–3) benchmarks for screening, diagnosis and early intervention (see Chapter 1) established by the JCIH also need to be a well-synchronized dance between birth hospitals, outpatient rescreening and diagnostic centers, amplification choice, device fitting and early intervention.[3–5] Difficulty accessing care at any of these points presents a bottleneck as intervention cannot occur until diagnosis has been completed.[6]

Barriers to timely diagnosis and intervention

In 2018, across the USA and its territories, an impressive 98.9% of live births received newborn hearing screening.[7] However, of the 1.6% of newborns who did not pass two-stage hearing screening in 2018, about 1 in 4 babies failed to receive timely diagnosis, and another 1 in 3 did not receive early intervention services for diagnosed hearing loss. Thus, only 49% of infants who had PHL met the 1–3–6 benchmarks to receive the benefits of EHDI.

Barriers that cause delays in timely diagnosis and may result in infants becoming lost to follow-up after failed newborn hearing screening are widespread in the USA.[8] Identified barriers to diagnosis and intervention include:[4,9,10]

- limited access to pediatric audiologists
- other medical conditions that may make follow up difficult
- middle ear fluid (MEF)
- mild or unilateral hearing loss
- family belief that the child is hearing adequately after observing his or her response to sounds in a familiar environment.

Nationally in the USA, lost-to-follow-up rates for UNHS vary from less than 5% in some states to more than 75% in others, due to systemic differences in EHDI programs across the country. Notably, wealthier states with majority White populations are achieving the 1–3–6 benchmarks at far higher rates than poorer or more rural states with bigger Black and Latinx populations. Children are at higher risk of being lost to follow-up at both the diagnosis and intervention stages if their mothers are non-White, less than 30 years old, covered by public insurance, have lower levels of maternal education, smoked during pregnancy, or reside in rural locations.[11–13] System-related bottlenecks and delays reported by rural families include poor communication of hearing screening results, difficulty in obtaining outpatient testing, inconsistencies in healthcare information from primary care providers, lack of local resources, insurance-related healthcare delays, and conflict with family and work responsibilities.[14]

Holte et al. (2012)[15] evaluated the factors that led to follow-up delays after newborn hearing screening in a study of 193 infants with hearing loss who had failed screening. Of the families who waited more than 3 months after the first diagnostic test for confirmation of hearing loss, the most common reason given by parents for the delay was the need for multiple diagnostic tests. Multiple audiology sessions are an inconvenience for parents, especially if there are transportation and scheduling issues. Most importantly, they may result in a delay before the child with hearing loss receives amplification and intervention services. Ideally, all the information necessary to either confirm normal hearing or to establish frequency-specific thresholds for each ear for initial hearing aid fitting should be obtained at the first audiology appointment following referral from newborn screening using protocols that include middle ear assessment, OAE testing, and frequency- and ear-specific ABR, including bone conduction testing.[5,16]

Middle ear fluid and conductive hearing loss

Difficulties in achieving a timely diagnosis occur for many reasons, but one of the most common is the presence of MEF that causes screening failure through transient CHL.[4,10,17] Delayed diagnosis because of coexistent MEF has been reported in 36% of infants with congenital or early-onset PHL.[18] Despite a relatively low likelihood of a child with a non-pass screen having PHL, primary care providers should never encourage watchful waiting, as delayed identification is detrimental for developmental outcomes.

Little is known about the natural history of CHL over the first year in newborns referred from UNHS relative to infants who pass hearing screening. Consequently, their management needs are unclear.[19] After birth, the middle ear is not immediately aerated, and may retain amniotic fluid and other debris. Vernix is also present in the newborn ear canal, obstructing 50% of the canal on average, and the amount of vernix is related to reduced middle ear transmission across frequencies.[20] Fluid or material such as amniotic fluid, mesenchyme or meconium in the newborn middle ear space has been reported in temporal bone and MRI studies,[21,22] and can affect both OAE and ABR testing. Histological studies have shown that amniotic fluid containing meconium may cause a foreign-body reaction in the middle ear that predisposes infants to later persistent or recurrent otitis media, explaining why failed newborn screening due to middle ear causes may predict later recurrent or chronic otitis media with effusion in infants.[23,24]

A common misconception is that middle ear function cannot be assessed at birth, and that MEF cannot be detected in newborns. In fact, wideband measures of newborn ears have been studied since the first measures reported by Keefe et al. (2000) in a large multisite study at four US sites.[25] The study showed that reflectance could assist in controlling false-positive outcomes resulting from poor probe seals in OAE testing. Many subsequent studies have found that using wideband absorbance testing or 1 kHz tympanometry is effective at detecting MEF that causes transient CHL. Referrals following OAE-based infant hearing screening are strongly associated with a finding of increased wideband absorbance, suggesting middle ear dysfunction at birth.[26,27] Wideband absorbance can be tested quickly if available on the equipment used for OAE screening, or at the time of diagnostic testing. Based on these wideband middle ear tests, an estimated 80–90% of distortion product OAE (DPOAE) screening referrals are due to transient outer or middle ear conditions.[26,27]

Newborns with poor absorbance at initial screening should be rescreened before discharge, because most middle ear problems are transient and resolve spontaneously. If absorbance and OAE or ABR tests are not passed at rescreening, referral to an otologist for ear examination could be suggested along with diagnostic testing. Newborns with normal absorbance and a 'refer' result for the hearing screen should be referred immediately, without further screening, to an audiologist for diagnostic testing because of the higher risk for PHL.[27]

Diagnosing the presence of middle ear fluid

A limited number of audiology clinics have expertise in the tests needed to confirm middle ear disease in newborns and wait times for referral appointments can be long. The necessary tests require a sleeping infant, and success rates decrease as the child's age increases. By 6 months of age, anesthesia or sedation is necessary for accurate diagnostic testing, which comes with health risks, increased parental anxiety and increased costs.[16]

Studies of newborn screening referrals have found that tympanostomy tube insertion is needed in one-third to one-half of cases with MEF to exclude underlying PHL.[28,29] In infants referred to a pediatric hospital from newborn screening, MEF was identified in 65%, and ventilation tubes were required in 35% of these infants before definitive diagnosis could be made.[28] Furthermore, 79% of infants without effusion were found to have PHL, whereas 11% of those with MEF had PHL. This highlights the importance of not assuming that MEF, if present, is always the cause of hearing loss.

Another study of screening failures found that 55% of infants had MEF and that 23% of these cases resolved spontaneously.[29] In the remaining infants, hearing normalized after tympanocentesis or placement of ventilation tubes, but only 69% of children had immediate resolution of normal hearing. The remaining 31% had a delayed return of hearing over several months, with a median of 4.8 months for all children combined.[29] This study demonstrates that surgery for MEF does not normalize hearing immediately.

Continued MEF and CHL in the first year have been reported in newborns who did not pass hearing screening.[30–32] There is a need to determine whether newborn MEF has a differential rate of resolution or natural history than fluid in older infants and children,[33] and whether intervention, such as myringotomy or ventilation tubes, is needed.

Reducing losses to follow-up

Families generally report a great desire to obtain timely hearing healthcare for their children[13] and express a willingness to use resources such as telemedicine to obtain that care.[14] Guidelines are available to help pediatric medical homecare providers ensure timely follow-up after newborn screening, diagnosis and intervention.[34] The JCIH and National Institute for Children's Health Quality (NICHQ) also recommend best practice steps and processes to reduce delays and bottlenecks and improve outcomes throughout the EHDI process (Figure 7.1).

An important proactive way to reduce losses to follow-up at the time of screening referral is to contact families quickly to schedule follow-up. Families may have only transient phone numbers and addresses, making it more difficult to reach them with increasing time after birth.[13] For this reason, it is best practice to proactively schedule follow-up before the infant leaves the birth hospital, rather than waiting for families to initiate follow-up later. States that report the lowest lost-to-follow-up rates use this practice.[35]

Another proactive approach is to provide convenient outpatient rescreening closer to home. An outpatient rescreening intervention study completed at women, infant and child (WIC) centers showed that about one-third of families reported barriers to obtaining follow-up services, especially lack of transportation or long distances from the diagnostic facility, lack of childcare, work or school scheduling conflicts, not having English as their first language and a lack of insurance coverage.[13] A positive outcome of this study was that providing convenient outpatient rescreening and parent education at WIC centers improved follow-up rates by about 70%.

Consistent counseling and education about the urgency of following up a non-pass screening as soon as possible are also essential.[5] Reasons cited by parents for delaying follow-up include being assured that the failed screening was likely caused by something other than PHL (such as MEF, an equipment problem or a cesarean delivery), believing that hearing could not be tested until the baby was older, or being advised to 'wait and see' if the baby responded to sound.

An overall important principle for success is collaboration and coordination between state agencies, hearing screening coordinators

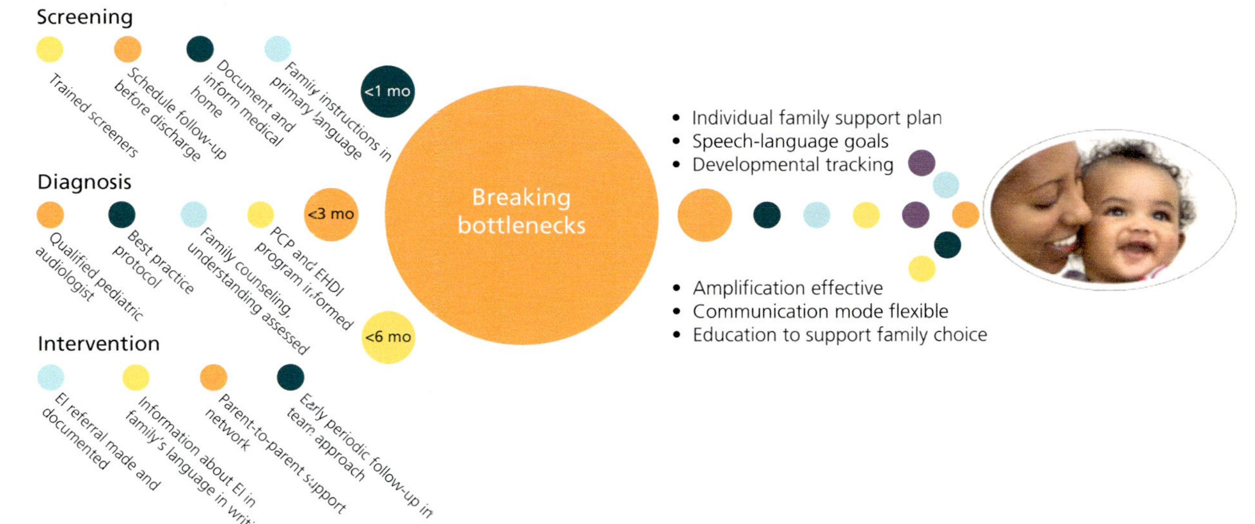

Figure 7.1 JCIH and NICHQ recommendations for best practice steps and processes to reduce losses to follow-up throughout the EHDI process, meet the EHDI 1–3–6 benchmarks and optimize outcomes for children identified with congenital PHL. EI, early intervention; mo, month; PCP, primary care provider.

at birth hospitals, pediatricians and other primary care providers, diagnostic audiologists, neonatologists and otolaryngologists.[5]

Further research is needed into how to best reduce loss to follow-up by providing coordinated care between birth hospitals and diagnostic centers. A major limitation to sustained improvement is funding and acceptance of the UNHS/EHDI model on a broader scale. Involving parents in shared decision-making to emphasize the importance of follow-up, and discuss the options for and barriers to follow-up, may improve adherence to recommendations.[33]

Key points – middle ear effusion and other barriers to timely diagnosis

- The presence of MEF causing transient CHL is one of the most common reasons for hearing screening failure.
- MEF, if present, is not necessarily the cause of PHL.
- Some of the barriers to achieving timely follow-up of infants who fail newborn hearing screening include difficulty in obtaining testing, distance to diagnostic facilities, the need for multiple diagnostic tests, scheduling conflicts (work, schooling) and lack of insurance coverage.
- Parents should be given consistent messages about the importance of timely follow-up and 'watchful waiting' should be discouraged.

References

1. Tomblin JB, Harrison M, Ambrose SE et al. Language outcomes in young children with mild to severe hearing loss. *Ear Hear* 2015;36(suppl 1): 76S–91S.
2. Ching TY. Is early intervention effective in improving spoken language outcomes of children with congenital hearing loss? *Am J Audiol* 2015;24:345–8.

3. Yoshinaga-Itano C, Sedey AL, Wiggin M, Chung W. Early hearing detection and vocabulary of children with hearing loss. *Pediatrics* 2017;14:e20162964.
4. Awad R, Oropeza J, Uhler KM. Meeting the Joint Committee on Infant Hearing standards in a large metropolitan children's hospital: barriers and next steps. *Am J Audiol* 2019;28:251–9.
5. Joint Committee on Infant Hearing. Year 2019 position statement: principles and guidelines for early hearing detection and intervention programs. *J Early Hear Detect Interv* 2019;4:1–44.
6. Spivak L, Sokol H. Beyond newborn screening: early diagnosis and management of hearing loss in infants. *Adv Neonatal Care* 2005;5:104–12.
7. Centers for Disease Control and Prevention. *Hearing loss in children: 2018 summary of CDC EHDI data*. 2018; www.cdc.gov/ncbddd/hearingloss/2018-data/01-data-summary.html, last accessed 6 June 2021.
8. Gaffney M, Green DR, Gaffney C. Newborn hearing screening and follow-up: are children receiving recommended services? *Public Health Rep* 2010;125:199–207.
9. Walker EA, Spratford M, Ambrose SE et al. Service delivery to children with mild hearing loss: current practice patterns and parent perceptions. *Am J Audiol* 2017;26:38–52.
10. Fitzpatrick EM, Cesconetto Dos Santos J, Grandpierre V, Whittingham J. Exploring reasons for late identification of children with early-onset hearing loss. *Int J Pediatr Otorhinolaryngol* 2017;100:160–7.
11. Zhang L, Links AR, Boss EF et al. Identification of potential barriers to timely access to pediatric hearing aids. *JAMA Otolaryngol Head Neck Surg* 2020;146:13–19.
12. Cunningham M, Thomson V, McKiever E et al. Infant, maternal, and hospital factors' role in loss to follow-up after failed newborn hearing screening. *Acad Pediatr* 2018;18:188–95.
13. Hunter LL, Meinzen-Derr J, Wiley S, et al. Influence of the WIC program on loss to follow-up for newborn hearing screening. *Pediatrics* 2016;138:e20154301.
14. Elpers J, Lester C, Shinn JB, Bush ML. Rural family perspectives and experiences with early infant hearing detection and intervention: a qualitative study. *J Community Health* 2016;41:226–33.
15. Holte L, Walker E, Oleson J et al. Factors influencing follow up to newborn hearing screening for infants who are hard of hearing. *Am J Audiol* 2012;21:163–74.

16. Sininger YS, Hunter LL, Hayes D et al. Evaluation of speed and accuracy of next-generation auditory steady state response and auditory brainstem response audiometry in children with normal hearing and hearing loss. *Ear Hear* 2018;39:1207–23.
17. Aithal S, Aithal V, Kei J, Driscoll C. Conductive hearing loss and middle ear pathology in young infants referred through a newborn universal hearing screening program in Australia. *J Am Acad Audiol* 2012;23:673–85.
18. Vartiainen E. Otitis media with effusion in children with congenital or early-onset hearing impairment. *J Otolaryngol* 2000;29:221–3.
19. Rosenfeld RM, Shin JJ, Schwartz SR et al. Clinical practice guideline: otitis media with effusion executive summary (update). *Otolaryngol Head Neck Surg* 2016;154:201–14.
20. Pitaro J, Al Masaoudi L, Motallebzadeh H et al. Wideband reflectance measurements in newborns: relationship to otoscopic findings. *Int J Pediatr Otorhinolaryngol* 2016;86:156–60.
21. Sano M, Kaga K, Mima K. MRI findings of the middle ear in infants. *Acta Otolaryngol* 2007;127:821–4.
22. Piza JE, Northrop CC, Eavey RD. Neonatal mesenchyme temporal bone study: typical receding pattern versus increase in Potter's sequence. *Laryngoscope* 1996;106:856–64.
23. Lilja M, Palva T, Ramsay H et al. Meconium contaminated amniotic fluid and infant otitis media. Is it a risk factor in children surviving aspiration and initial distress of respiration? *Int J Pediatr Otorhinolaryngol* 2006;70:655–62.
24. Palva T, Northrop C, Ramsay H. Foreign body neonatal otitis media in infants. *Otol Neurotol* 2001;22:433–43.
25. Keefe DH, Folsom RC, Gorga MP et al. Identification of neonatal hearing impairment: ear-canal measurements of acoustic admittance and reflectance in neonates. *Ear Hear* 2000; 21:443–61.
26. Sanford CA, Keefe DH, Liu Y-W et al. Sound-conduction effects on distortion-product otoacoustic emission screening outcomes in newborn infants: test performance of wideband acoustic transfer functions and 1-kHz tympanometry. *Ear Hear* 2009;30:635–52.
27. Hunter LL, Feeney MP, Lapsley Miller JA et al. Wideband reflectance in newborns: normative regions and relationship to hearing-screening results. *Ear Hear* 2010;31:599–610.
28. Boone RT, Bower CM, Martin PF. Failed newborn hearing screens as presentation for otitis media with effusion in the newborn population. *Int J Pediatr Otorhinolaryngol* 2005;69:393–7.

29. Boudewyns A, Declau F, Van den Ende J et al. Otitis media with effusion: an underestimated cause of hearing loss in infants. *Otol Neurotol* 2011;32:799–804.
30. Doyle KJ, Kong YY, Strobel K et al. Neonatal middle ear effusion predicts chronic otitis media with effusion. *Otol Neurotol* 2004;25:318–22.
31. Pereira PK, Azevedo MF, Testa JR. Conductive impairment in newborn who failed the newborn hearing screening. *Braz J Otorhinolaryngol* 2010;76: 347–54.
32. Chen JL. Newborn hearing screening may predict Eustachian tube dysfunction. *Int J Pediatr Otorhinolaryngol* 2015;79:2099–103.
33. Rosenfeld RM, Shin JJ, Schwartz SR et al. Clinical practice guideline: otitis media with effusion (update). *Otolaryngol Head Neck Surg* 2016;154(1 suppl):S1–S41.
34. American Academy of Pediatrics Task Force for Improving Newborn Hearing Screening, Diagnosis and Intervention. Early hearing detection and intervention (EHDI) guidelines for pediatric medical home providers. https://health.utah.gov/cshcn/pdf/EHDI/EHDI%20Guidelines%20for%20Pediatricians.pdf, last accessed 9 June 2022.
35. Russ SA, Hanna D, DesGeorges J, Forsman I. Improving follow-up to newborn hearing screening: a learning-collaborative experience. *Pediatrics* 2010; 126(suppl 1):S59–69.

Further reading and resources

American Academy of Pediatrics. Early hearing detection and intervention. www.aap.org/en/patient-care/early-hearing-detection-and-intervention, last accessed 9 June 2022.

Centers for Disease Control and Prevention. Hearing loss in children. www.cdc.gov/ncbddd/hearingloss/index.html, last accessed 1 July 2021.

National Institute for Children's Health Equality. Improving follow-up after newborn hearing screening: an action kit for audiologists. http://trigonroad.com/ak/Improving%20Follow%20Up%20Audiology%20Guide%20-%20Final%20Draft%20to%20Editor%201.20.pdf, last accessed 1 July 2021.

Healthy Children.org. Newborn hearing screening FAQs. www.healthychildren.org/English/ages-stages/baby/Pages/Purpose-of-Newborn-Hearing-Screening.aspx, last accessed 1 July 2021.

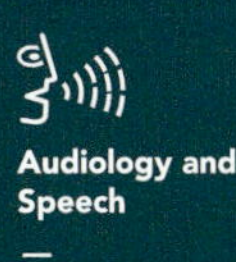

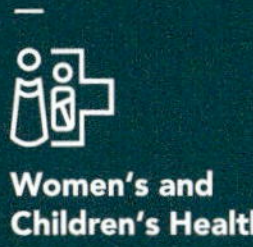

8 Data management systems for newborn hearing screening programs

Adrian C Davis, Christine Yoshinaga-Itano
and Gwen Carr

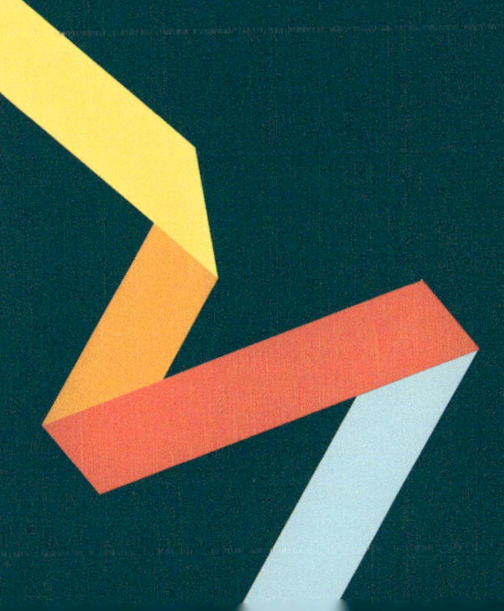

HEALTHCARE

This chapter discusses the data needed to implement, sustain and evaluate newborn hearing screening programs and the development of data management systems. Because of the cost of developing an EHDI program, funders expect regular reports about progress toward achieving the program's goals and unless there is a comprehensive data management system, it is not possible to determine what progress is being made. Many countries that offer UNHS/EHDI are unable to report statistics about the quality of their programs. As a result, we know little about the prevalence of pediatric hearing loss throughout the world and we do not know how young children with hearing loss are being supported or developing.

Data and data management

For the effective quality assurance of EHDI programs, it is essential to have accurate and timely data. Data are characteristics or information, usually numerical, that are collected through observation.

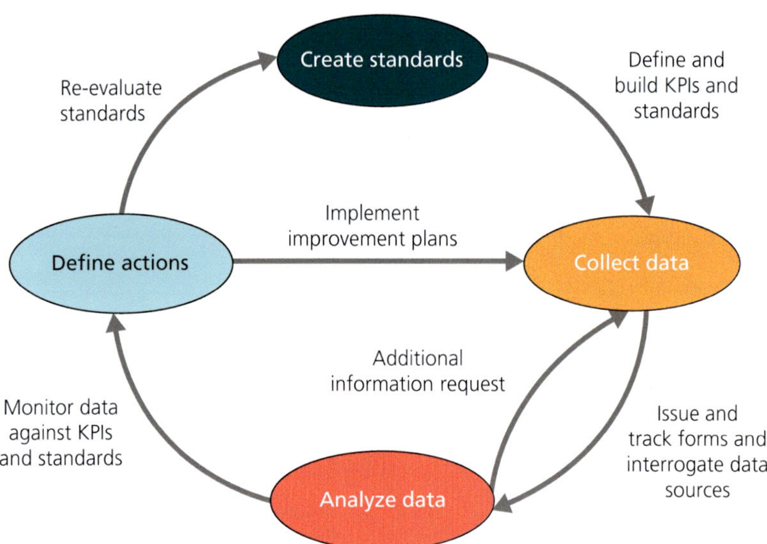

Figure 8.1 Stages in developing and sustaining a data management system. KPI, key performance indicator.

In a more technical sense, data are a set of values covering qualitative or quantitative variables about one or more persons or objects, while a datum (singular of data) is a single value of a single variable.

Data management systems create standards, define actions, and collect and analyze data in a continuous manner (Figure 8.1). They can interrogate data to analyze a program's function, assess its quality, and track and monitor progress toward its goals (Table 8.1).

There are, broadly speaking, two types of data needed within a management system. These are:

- data that are used to ensure the program runs correctly, tracking babies, families and screening outcomes
- data that can be used to indicate the quality and outcomes of the program.

Some data will be countable and some will reflect the timing and order of events; other data will concern the quality of the service offered (Table 8.2). Quantitative data can give insights into patient journeys and the continuity or discontinuity experienced by families and children. Qualitative data help program providers understand how parents felt about their experiences with UNHS/EHDI.

TABLE 8.1

Using data to monitor performance

Data management systems can help answer questions such as:

- Are referred infants obtaining an audiological diagnostic evaluation to confirm hearing loss?
- Is the audiological diagnostic evaluation conducted by 3 months of age?
- Are the infants who are confirmed as DHH referred and enrolled in early intervention services?
- Are the parents of infants who are confirmed as DHH informed about amplification technology and when?
- What percentage of infants are fitted with amplification technology and when?
- What are the developmental outcomes (at school entrance age) of the children who are confirmed as DHH?

TABLE 8.2

Examples of data collected for management systems

Countable data

- How many babies were born?
- How many babies were screened?
- How many babies were then referred for assessment?
- How many babies completed audiological diagnostic evaluation?
- How many children who are DHH were identified?
- How many infants received specialist medical evaluation?
- How many families were offered (and accepted) amplification technology?
- How many families received supportive early intervention services?

Data reflecting timing and order of events

- At what age was the screening completed, relative to birth?
- At what age was the audiological diagnostic evaluation completed?
- At what ages were medical and genetic diagnostic evaluations conducted?
- When was early intervention offered and what was the date of enrollment/age of the child?

Other relevant data

- How was consent sought?
- How was the screen carried out?
- How was the result of the screen communicated?
- How were next steps communicated?
- How was audiological diagnostic evaluation handled – who made the appointment and when was the appointment made?
- How was the medical evaluation handled? Who made the the appointment and when?
- Were families offered technology and informed about their rights and choices? How equitable is access to technology socioeconomically
  - for instance, is technology available only for those with financial resources?

CONTINUED

TABLE 8.2 CONTINUED

Examples of data collected for management systems

- From the family's perspective, was early intervention provided in a timely manner and did they receive information and develop skills necessary to support their child's development?
- How knowledgeable were participants about the events/actions/activities around the rationale and process in EHDI – for example:
  - the overall screening process
  - the referral process
  - the audiological diagnostic evaluation, medical and genetic assessments
  - the early intervention referral and services
- Did the process cause undue stress; were the families supported throughout the process?

The goals for a successful EHDI program are meeting the 1–3–6 benchmarks (see Chapter 1) and demonstrating development within the normal range for the majority of infants identified as DHH. Data collected for the data management system therefore need to be able to document screening by 1 month, identification by 3 months and enrollment in early intervention services by 6 months (and amplification device fitting within 1 month of diagnosis).

The data collected need to be uniformly collated, with agreement from the outset on what data are required, the definitions for each data point, and the coding and analysis procedures for reporting. For instance, what defines when a screen has occurred? Does 'screen completion' refer to the screen before hospital discharge or, if there is an outpatient screen, are those data also recorded? Is completion of the screen defined as the completion of both the in-hospital and outpatient screen?

EHDI systems develop over time and data provide both the impetus to improve and the insight to know where to focus.

Setting up a data management system

Just as EHDI systems develop over time, so too do data management systems and, at each stage, the capability of the system becomes more sophisticated (Table 8.3).

TABLE 8.3

Functionality checklist for data management systems

Basic/emerging systems

Is the data management system able to fulfill the following requirements?

- Identify all newborns eligible for newborn hearing screening:
  - Does a separate system need to be developed or is there the option of merging with existing newborn data management systems?
- Assure the ability to:
  - document whether a screen has occurred and the result of the screen
  - track and document whether infants who are referred to follow-up attend outpatient screening and diagnostic audiological evaluation
  - track results of diagnostic audiological evaluation and age at identification
  - record referral to early intervention services and age at initiation of early intervention services
  - record referral and receipt of family-to-family support
  - fit amplification device and report age at fitting in infants diagnosed as DHH
  - document language, speech, socioemotional and literacy developmental outcomes compared with cognitive development
  - report the number and proportion of children who meet the 1–3–6 or 1–2–3 benchmarks
  - report the number and proportion of children who achieve age-appropriate development in all developmental areas
- Determine availability of family-to-family support and DHH leaders
- Embed data analysis and reporting as a core element of the program
- Use data to ensure ongoing monitoring of program performance

CONTINUED

TABLE 8.3 CONTINUED

Emerging/intermediate systems
Is the data management system able to fulfill the following requirements? • Determine accomplishment of all criteria on the basic/emerging checklist • Focus on expansion and maintaining quality of pilot UNHS/EHDI programs • Embed data analysis and reporting as a core element of the program, if this has not yet been done • Use data to ensure ongoing monitoring of program performance, if this has not yet been done • Document the provision of parent-to-parent support and parental involvement in system development and implementation • Document the provision of family-centered early intervention services • Document family access to DHH leadership networks and the involvement of individuals who are DHH in system development and implementation • Document longitudinal developmental outcomes of identified children • Document professional training and quality assurance progress monitoring
Advanced/mature systems
Is the data management system able to fulfill the following requirements? • Embed data analysis and reporting as a core element of the program, if this has not yet been implemented • Use data to ensure ongoing monitoring of program performance, if this has not been implemented, and make links to other newborn screening programs • Support the quality assurance of a program and its continuous improvement • Enable reporting of child and family journies and links to outcomes

CONTINUED

TABLE 8.3 CONTINUED

Functionality checklist for data management systems

Advanced/mature systems *(cont'd)*
• Chart progress for improvement of adherence to best practice standards for screening referral rates, follow-up rates, diagnostic evaluation protocols, amplification fit protocols and early intervention quality
• Document enrollment in family-centered early intervention services
• Analyze data on developmental monitoring every 6 months and initiate program development protocols and training based on outcomes
• Provide data to support calls to mandate early intervention by law or regulations to assure quality

Alternatives to formal data management systems. There are a number of strategies that can be used in situations where a formal data management system does not exist. On the smallest of scales, it is possible to begin with a paper system. In other cases, a possible strategy is to identify existing data management systems – such as birth registries or records of immunizations, genetic/metabolic screening and well-baby checks – and collaborate with these systems. Data should be analyzed after 3, 6, 9 and 12 months and action taken if the data do not meet expectations or aspirations. Data should also be gathered to assess whether the action made a difference.

Assuring quality

Quality management and progress assessment is a cyclical process (Figure 8.2). Data must be collected from multiple agencies (Figure 8.3) for quality management purposes, and the ability to interrogate data from both internal and external sources facilitates a holistic approach to a quality management framework that focuses on the interface and interaction between the multiple agencies involved in UNHS/EHDI services. Establishing explicit assurance criteria allows for consistent monitoring and evaluation of the services being offered.

Advanced data management systems offer the ability to automatically generate many different outputs, including standard

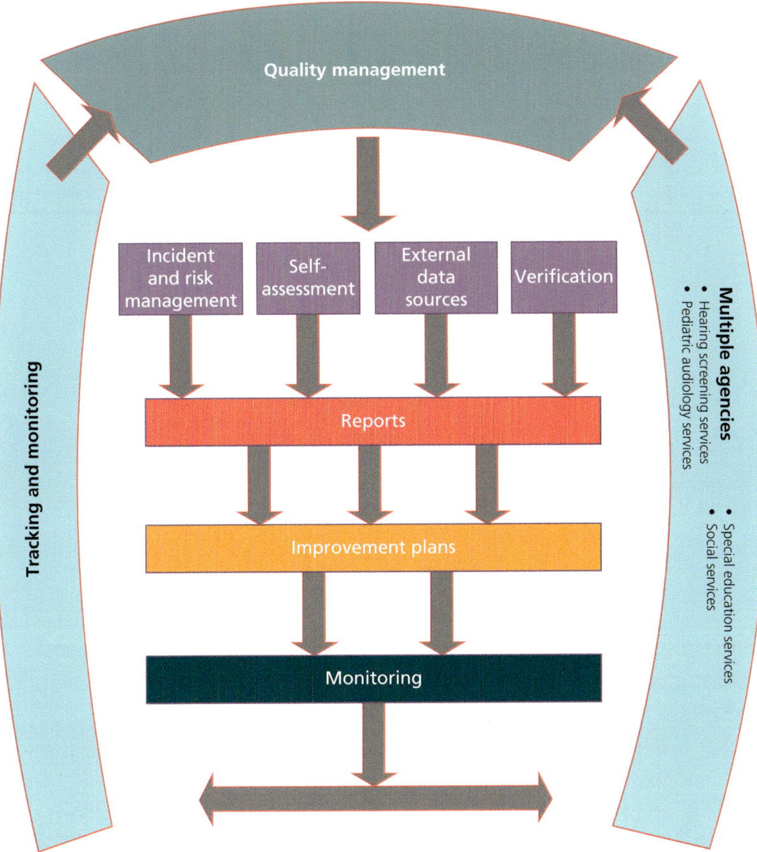

Figure 8.2 Quality management and progress monitoring process for a UNHS/EHDI program.

reports, graphs and documents. Automated monitoring of performance and trends, underpinned by escalation procedures, allows earlier and better-informed decision-making when an issue is identified, while automated monitoring of the delivery of an improvement plan can encourage proactivity in its implementation.

Standardized reporting across different sites involved in UNHS/EHDI creates consistency in outputs, increasing confidence that reports are fair and thorough. It also facilitates automatic

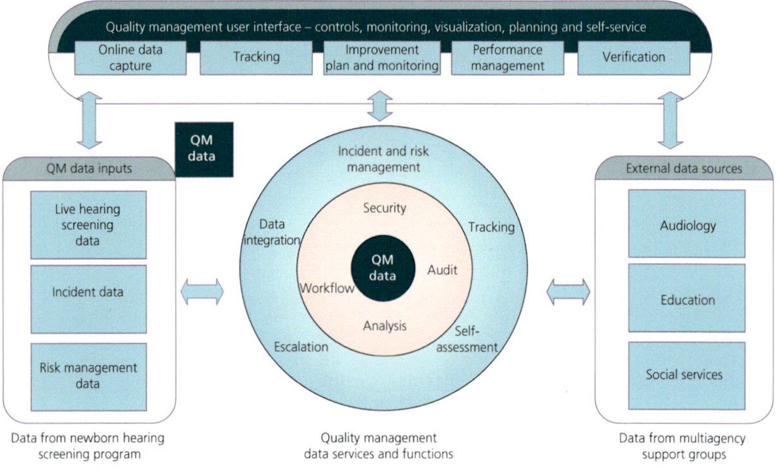

Figure 8.3 Sources of data for quality management (QM) of a UNHS/EHDI program.

benchmarking of performance across sites and the sharing of good working practices. Sharing data across screening networks can help optimize the delivery of UNHS/EHDI programs.

Key points – data management systems for newborn hearing screening programs

- Data management systems provide vital information to help determine progress toward achieving the goals of a UNHS/EHDI program.
- The collection and analysis of data to inform improvement is an ongoing, cyclical process.
- Data can be an indicator of whether a program is functioning correctly as well as of its quality and outcomes.
- As data management systems develop, their capabilities become increasingly sophisticated and can be used to support quality assurance and continuous development of a UNHS/EHDI program.

Further reading and resources

Centers for Disease Control. Early hearing detection and intervention information system (EHDI-IS) functional standards. www.cdc.gov/ncbddd/hearingloss/ehdi-is-functional-standards.html, last accessed 9 June 2022.

Commercially available data management systems

www.necsws.com/health-screening-software/

www.ozsystems.com

www.hitrack.org/

https://newborncare.natus.com/products-services/newborn-care-products/hearing-screening/audble-litedesktop

https://newborncare.natus.com/products-services/newborn-care-products/tracking-follow/neometrics-data-management

www.ntst.com/solutions/by-capability/electronic-health-records

www.mednax.com/solutions/services/newbornhearingscreenservices/

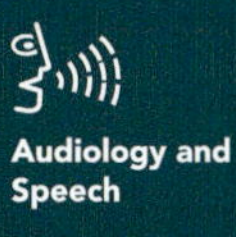

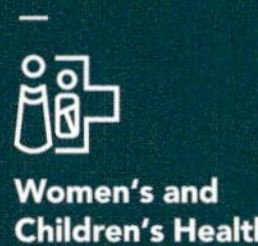

9 Establishing UNHS/EHDI programs

Doris R Lewis, Christine Yoshinaga-Itano, Adrian C Davis and Gwen Carr

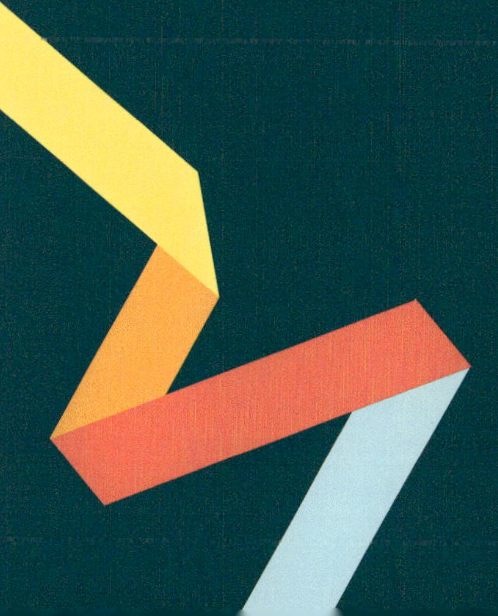

HEALTHCARE

Newborn hearing screening is the only strategy that enables population-based early identification of and intervention for infants with congenital PHL. Successful EHDI programs are part of a system of care that begins with neonatal hearing screening and then transitions through follow-up by audiological diagnostic assessment to subsequent enrollment into early intervention programs. This system of care requires many factors to be considered and UNHS programs must be developed according to evidence-based practice. Failure to attend to critical components of the system, whether that be diagnostic audiology capability, amplification, family-centered early intervention services (FCEI), parent-to-parent support, DHH leadership or developmental monitoring of children, can result in failure to accomplish the 1–3–6 benchmarks of the EHDI system (see Chapter 1) and thus reduce the likelihood that infants and children who are DHH achieve developmental milestones similar to their peers who are hearing.

How and when should infants be screened?

The JCIH recommends that evidence-based hearing screening protocols should result in no more than 4% of screened infants being referred on for diagnostic evaluation.[1] Different protocols are in use around the world, and referral rates are related to age at screening, test technology and the number of steps used in the protocol.[1,2]

Evidence suggests that all screening technologies (aABR only, OAE only and OAE followed by aABR) can be effective and with the appropriate protocol can result in referral rates under 4%.[1] The use of aABR alone has a significantly lower referral rate (average 0.8%) than OAE alone (5–22%), but runs the risk of missing infants with milder hearing loss. A double screen with both aABR and OAE can identify 24% more infants with hearing loss.[1,3] Using aABR assessment after OAE screening does require a second test, but referral rates can be lowered to 1–2%.[4,5] Repeated screenings with OAE have been used to significantly reduce referral rates when screening infants who are older than 72 hours[6] but repeated screening of only the 'refers' also increases the risk of missed hearing loss.

The referral rate can also depend on the age of the newborn at screening. Ideally, a UNHS program should offer screening in birth hospitals, but when this is not possible, screening should occur within the first month of life. A recent study has analyzed referral rates by age as reported by 23 different regions.[2] The referral rate when OAE was performed within 24 hours following birth was 6–22% with one or two OAE tests. This fell to 2–15% when the newborn was older than 24 hours, and to 4% for babies older than 72 hours. Referral rates averaged 2.1% after repeated screening using OAE before hospital discharge.[2]

The study also analyzed referral rates when OAE testing was followed by aABR after a baby did not pass the OAE screen. Overall, this resulted in a 1.7% referral rate.[2] Lower referral rates can result in better access to subsequent diagnostic audiological testing and reduced loss to follow-up, but also a higher probability that hearing loss may be missed.

Infants with risk indicators in the NICU should undergo aABR screening because of the high prevalence of hearing loss and ANSD among this population, which would be undetected with OAE screening.[1] Diagnostic audiological evaluation for referred infants in the NICU can then be carried out before hospital discharge, ensuring that intervention can begin as quickly as possible.

Behavioral screening of infants in the first year of life, such as distraction screening, should not be used because of high false-positive rates, leading to unnecessary hearing assessments.[1] Additionally, behavioral screening is only possible after 6 months of age when children begin to demonstrate a conditioned head-turn response. Using behavioral screening would therefore make it impossible to achieve the EHDI 1–3–6 benchmarks.

Protocols for UNHS programs should therefore be designed with the ability to record and report rates of referral to diagnostic testing and the subsequent diagnosis. Low rates of false-positive and false-negative results with any specific protocol or technology are necessary, along with high sensitivity, specificity and positive predictive value. These statistics establish the quality of the UNHS program in this first stage of neonatal hearing healthcare.

Planning a screening program

To decide whether there is capacity to begin a UNHS program, it is important to determine what resources are already available and what screening protocols, equipment, personnel, training of personnel and education for families are needed for the program being developed.

Each decision has specific ramifications for costs, the number of personnel required, the effectiveness of the screening program and the success of follow through, leading ultimately to optimal developmental outcomes for the infants identified as DHH.[1,7]

Current resources. The current availability of relevant resources, including both personnel and equipment, must be assessed at the outset of developing any new public health initiative to help inform future procurement needs. The presence of any existing form of hearing screening (for example, targeted screening in the NICU, or distraction behavioral screening after 6 months of age), the number of infants already being screened, and the number of dedicated personnel should be identified and the data management program evaluated (see Chapter 8).

The number of live births each year in each birthing hospital (by region, state and country as a whole) will inform human resource and infrastructure requirements and play a significant role in the choice of technology and determination of the number of pieces of screening equipment required.

Financial readiness. Sufficient financial support makes a program sustainable. In higher-income countries, government funding for equipment purchase and data management systems has typically been provided. In low- and middle-income countries, programs may be established initially using funding obtained through charitable organizations or non-governmental organizations. Equipment as well as personnel costs must be considered.

A further consideration is whether the UNHS program will be offered free to families or at a cost. Some hospitals build the cost of screening into the birthing cost. In higher-income countries, socialized medical systems or insurance companies cover the cost of screening, although uninsured individuals may have to pay the cost themselves. Some low- and middle-income countries charge families for the screen.

Public, parent and professional education. Public health initiatives such as UNHS must be supported by a means of educating the public, parents and healthcare professionals about the importance of the screening program. It is vital that all those involved understand why the screening program is being initiated and so opportunities to inform and educate must be identified. If information about public issues or healthcare initiatives is already shared with the public, there may be existing routes by which awareness of a screening program can be raised before the program itself is implemented.

It is also important to consider the public's attitude to identifying disability in newborns and young children and whether there are societal barriers to doing so. Cultural values and belief systems influence acceptance of a UNHS program and these issues should be addressed in the education program that prepares the public for the initiative.

Opportunities to inform and educate expectant mothers about the importance of newborn hearing screening may arise during their pregnancy and, typically, information about screening is provided during prenatal care. All personnel who interact with expectant mothers and with mothers during and after delivery should receive information and training about the hearing screening program.

Recruitment and training. All healthcare personnel involved in the UNHS program will need to be trained. It may be feasible for existing staff, such as maternity nurses, to be trained to undertake screening if they have the capacity to take on this task. Alternatively, a new workforce may need to be recruited, with screening being regarded as a specialized role. Audiologists/otolaryngologists are needed to oversee the hearing screening program.[8]

Those who carry out the hearing screening will need to learn how to operate and troubleshoot the equipment, and how to record and report data according to the protocols developed. They must also be trained to provide information to families before and after the screen. Personnel can be trained on typical 'scripts' that can be used to provide information to families for both the infants who pass the screening and those who are referred for additional testing. Both the screener and the physicians who provide postnatal care should emphasize the importance of follow-up. A system of providing appointments for parents whose child requires rescreening and those who require referral to audiological diagnostic evaluations should be identified and all pertinent personnel should be aware of these procedures.

Equipment considerations include the type of technology and the number of systems required as well as the locations needing the equipment and the specifications for screening, diagnostics, hearing aid fitting and supply of services.

In addition to determining the amount of hearing screening equipment required, it is also essential to ensure that there are sufficient diagnostic audiological centers with the appropriate equipment available. Furthermore, amplification technology, often the first step of intervention, requires specific equipment for hearing aid fitting.

The different types of neonatal facility and the number of infants in each type will also play a role in informing the choice of equipment. Infants in NICUs, for instance, should always be screened with aABR equipment to identify those with ANSD who would be missed if they were screened by OAE screening.

Technology will sometimes need repair, meaning that back-up equipment is also required to ensure that the screening program can be maintained in these instances.

Overall, UNHS programs must determine the cost of the equipment and of the personnel needed to operate it, consider the types of hearing loss missed by different screening technologies, the likelihood of loss to follow-up, the need to keep the referral rate to diagnostic evaluations below 4%, and the likelihood of meeting EHDI 1–3–6 benchmarks when making technology choices.

Screening location. Many birthing hospitals will discharge newborns within 24 hours if they do not require specialized care. As discussed above, infants screened within 24 hours of birth should be assessed by aABR and this should be factored in to equipment considerations. A further consideration is whether hospital personnel should be available to carry out screening 24 hours per day. If infants might be missed if screening is conducted only during the regular working day, there needs to be a system to track those who have not had in-hospital screening.

Likewise, infants in a NICU may be transferred to neonatal care facilities when their health status stabilizes and may or may not have completed the infant hearing screening before transfer. A tracking system should be in place to ensure that all these infants are screened and that they will receive follow-up screening or diagnostic evaluation after they are transferred. It is highly recommended that all high-risk babies have their hearing monitored as late onset of hearing loss can arise in some circumstances.

If infants are not typically born in hospitals, or if babies go home without being screened for any reason and it is not easy for their parents to bring them back for screening, other opportunities to carry out screening can be considered (Table 9.1). Again, the number of these settings will determine the amount and type of equipment required. The efficacy of screening in these other settings has not yet been evaluated and, in all cases, the question of cost in comparison to hospital screening will arise.

Data management. Regardless of whether screening takes place in hospital or in another setting, stable, reliable internet connectivity

TABLE 9.1

Alternative screening opportunities and considerations

- Hearing screening at home (this must take account of both logistics and cultural acceptability)
- Hearing screening in coordination with other universal newborn/postnatal screening programs, such as blood spot, heart, eye, hip:
  - Is the non-hearing screen a one-stage or two-stage process (would repeated hearing screening be feasible if needed)?
  - Is the data management system for non-hearing screening a potential management system for EHDI data?
- Hearing screening in coordination with a childhood vaccination program:
  - When and where do vaccinations take place?
  - Is the data management system a potential management system for UNHS/EHDI data?
- Hearing screening at postnatal healthcare/well-baby clinics:
  - At what intervals and where does the healthcare take place?
  - How many clinics are there?
  - What proportion of mothers and infants attend well-baby clinics?
  - Do the clinics offer the potential for a UNHS program or second hearing screening?

is essential for electronic data management systems. Personnel to provide IT support are also vital for sustainable data management systems. The following additional factors must be considered.

- Is there an existing data management system that the hearing screening results could be stored in and managed from, or is a dedicated system needed to store and manage the data?
- Does the data management system have sufficient fields to store all the screening results or just the latest test results?
- Who can access the data in the data management system to streamline the follow-up, if needed?
- Are there measures for privacy protection?
- What is the data backup protocol?
- What is the data monitoring protocol to assure reliability and validity of the screening process?

Consent for medical services is also a consideration during the planning stage for a new public health initiative. The requirements for consent for medical procedures will vary from government to government. Some will require consent from every family for screening, while others will assume consent unless a family actively declines the screen. This latter option usually results in higher levels of screening than the opt-in option. Verbal consent has also been found to have high opt-in rates.

Further considerations for screening programs

Target group. Some children with hearing loss will be missed with all screening technology.[1] Screening programs must determine which children are their priority for identification – for example, children with moderate-to-severe to profound hearing loss, children with ANSD or children with mild hearing loss – and select the most appropriate screening technology.[1] As discussed above, the disadvantage of screening first with OAE technology is that children with ANSD will be missed and these losses, although rare in the well-baby nursery, can have a significant impact on development. However, OAE technology identifies more newborns with mild hearing loss that have been missed by aABR technology.[2]

Preterm infants should have their hearing screened through aABR screening protocols because of the higher probability of ANSD among infants in NICUs, although pass/refer outcomes are based on average responses for term babies. For this reason, calibration and normative data must be provided by manufacturers to screening program coordinators, who in turn should inform those carrying out the screening of the potential of different devices in relation to the ages of children to be tested. When the equipment is not appropriate, hearing should be tested with conventional ABR equipment either in hearing diagnostic clinics with pediatric audiology experts, or before hospital discharge. Very premature infants are typically screened close to discharge and diagnostic audiological evaluation before discharge ensures the earliest enrollment in intervention for those that require it.

Best practice can be achieved if the personnel carrying out screening are trained and receive all the required information from UNHS coordinators and equipment manufacturers. Such training should cover the protocols to be applied, newborn/child state (asleep/awake/mildly sedated) during screening, observation of the ear canal, communication with parents, understanding the need to achieve benchmarks for test-retest, the multiple stages and steps in the protocol, the implementation of quality assurance procedures and the use of appropriate statistics.[1]

Setting higher benchmarks. The JCIH 2019 position statement reinforces the need to achieve the EHDI 1–3–6 benchmarks for all infants with hearing loss, except for those who remain in a NICU for longer than 1 month.[1] For sites that achieve these benchmarks, the JCIH recommends the 1–2–3 benchmarks (see Chapter 1). Regardless of the target, achieving either EHDI 1–3–6 or EHDI 1–2–3 benchmarks requires well-established protocols for screening, diagnosis and enrollment in intervention to create an integrated system for neonatal hearing healthcare.[1]

Parental anxiety. There is always a concern about parental anxiety caused by referral/failure in newborn hearing screening. However, when UNHS programs follow evidence-based practice, parental anxiety has been found to be comparable to the general anxiety associated with the birth of a child.[9] High referral rates can cause unnecessary emotional distress and programs that fail to provide general information to parents/families about the rationale for hearing screening and the importance of follow-up have been associated with higher levels of parental anxiety.[9–15]

Repeated testing of only those newborns who have a 'refer' result on first screening, in order to obtain a higher pass response rate, can result in reducing referrals to a very low rate, with the risk that hearing loss can be missed. The JCIH therefore emphasizes that no more than two high-quality hospital-based tests should be performed before a newborn is discharged, and one high-quality screen as an outpatient retest. The infant must be quiet, mostly sleeping, with low noise in the environment during testing.[1]

The 2019 JCIH position statement refers to many other issues around neonatal hearing healthcare, from screening through to intervention. For this reason, programs interested in establishing a UNHS system should read the full document.[1]

Key points – establishing UNHS/EHDI programs

- Newborn hearing screening must be implemented to achieve early identification and intervention for infants with congenital PHL.
- Well babies can be screened with either aABR or OAE technology.
- Behavioral tests are not recommended as they give high levels of false-positive and false-negative outcomes and cannot be administered in the newborn period.
- Referral rates for diagnostic testing should be lower than 4% of newborns screened; depending on the technology used, referral rates can be less than 1–2% in well babies when evidence-based protocols are followed.
- All infants in the NICU should be screened with aABR to identify those with ANSD.
- A double technology screen (aABR followed by OAE) for infants in the NICU may be the most effective in identifying the highest proportion of infants with hearing loss.
- Trained professionals and best practices will increase the likelihood of achieving optimal outcomes for child development.

References

1. Joint Committee on Infant Hearing. 2019 position statement: principles and guidelines for early hearing detection and intervention programs. *J Early Hear Detect Interv* 2019;4:1–44.
2. Mackey AR, Bussé AML, Hoeve HLJ et al; EUS€REEN Foundation. Assessment of hearing screening programmes across 47 countries or regions II: coverage, referral, follow-up and detection rates from newborn hearing screening. *Int J Audiol* 2021;60:831–40.
3. Levit Y, Himmelfarb M, Dollberg S. Sensitivity of the automated auditory brainstem response in neonatal hearing screening. *Pediatrics* 2015;136:e641–7.
4. Lin HC, Shu MT, Lee KS et al. Reducing false positives in newborn hearing screening program: how and why. *Otol Neurotol* 2007;28:788–92.
5. van Dyk M, Swanepoel de W, Hall JW 3rd. Outcomes with OAE and AABR screening in the first 48 h—implications for newborn hearing screening in developing countries. *Int J Pediatr Otorhinolaryngol* 2015;79:1034–40.
6. Akinpelu OV, Peleva E, Funnell WR, Daniel SJ. Otoacoustic emissions in newborn hearing screening: a systematic review of the effects of different protocols on test outcomes. *Int J Pediatr Otorhinolaryngol* 2014;78:711–7.
7. Joint Committee on Infant Hearing. Year 2007 position statement: principles and guidelines for early hearing detection and intervention programs. *Pediatrics* 2007;120:898–921.
8. Thomson V, Yoshinaga-Itano C. The role of audiologists in assuring follow-up to outpatient screening in early hearing detection and intervention systems. *Am J Audiol* 2018;27:283–93.
9. Tueller SJ, White KR. Maternal anxiety associated with newborn hearing screening. *J Early Hear Detect Interv* 2016;1:87–92.
10. Watkin PM, Baldwin M, Dixon R, Beckman A. Maternal anxiety and attitudes to universal neonatal hearing screening. *Br J Audiol* 1998;32:27–37.
11. Crockett R, Wright AJ, Uus K et al. Maternal anxiety following newborn hearing screening: the moderating role of knowledge. *J Med Screen* 2006;13:20–5.

12. Crockett R, Baker H, Uus K et al. Maternal anxiety and satisfaction following infant hearing screening: a comparison of the health visitor distraction test and newborn hearing screening. *J Med Screen* 2005;12:78–82.
13. Vohr BR, Letourneau KS, McDermott C. Maternal worry about neonatal hearing screening. *J Perinatol* 2001;21:15–20.
14. Kolski C, Le Driant B, Lorenzo P et al. Early hearing screening: what is the best strategy? *Int J Pediatr Otorhinolaryngol* 2007;71:1055–60.
15. Khairi MDM, Rafidah KN, Affizal A et al. Anxiety of the mothers with referred baby during universal newborn hearing screening. *Int J Pediatr Otorhinolaryngol* 2011;75:513–17.

Further reading and resources

Joint Committee on Infant Hearing. Position statements. www.jcih.org/posstatemts.htm, last accessed 9 June 2022.

UK Government. NHS newborn hearing screening programme (NHSP): detailed information. www.gov.uk/topic/population-screening-programmes/newborn-hearing, last accessed 9 June 2022.

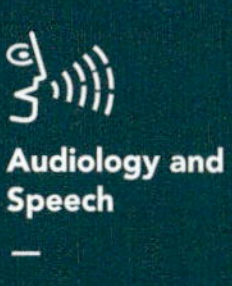

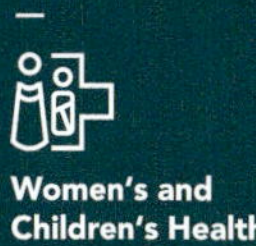

10 Pediatric diagnostic audiology

Doris R Lewis and Christine Yoshinaga-Itano

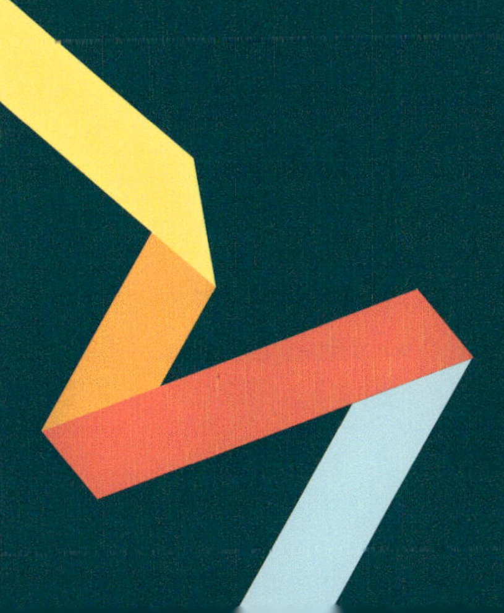

HEALTHCARE

Quality EHDI systems require accurate diagnosis of hearing loss in newborns referred from UNHS. The earlier a child can be confirmed as DHH, the sooner early intervention services can be provided. Infants with hearing loss should be referred to early intervention services even if the type of hearing loss (sensorineural, conductive, mixed) is still to be determined, as initiating early intervention services within the first 3 months of life is associated with significantly better developmental outcomes for children who are DHH.[1–3]

There are multiple factors to be considered in establishing a pediatric audiological diagnostic service (Table 10.1). Appropriate knowledge, skills and access to the necessary equipment are essential to prevent inaccurate diagnoses of hearing loss.[4–6] In the USA, audiological diagnosis in infants is the sole purview of the pediatric audiologist, while in other countries there may be an equivalent professional (for example, an audiological physician) who performs early childhood audiological diagnostic evaluations. Only through consultation with such an audiologist can accurate diagnosis occur, and early intervention for the infant and family be assured. It is incumbent on any audiologist who lacks the experience or equipment needed to conduct audiological evaluation of infants to refer on to audiology centers where timely and comprehensive evaluation can be accomplished.

Audiological diagnostic evaluation in infants

Audiological diagnosis in infants must be conducted in a timely manner, optimally by 2–3 months of age.[4–7] This earlier age facilitates the diagnostic process as infants are more likely to sleep for prolonged periods, allowing adequate time for an assessment to be carried out without sedation. In children with special health needs, a delay in diagnosing hearing loss may be unavoidable because of the need for other health-/time-urgent diagnostic and treatment procedures. However, every effort should be made to minimize the delays and, when feasible, audiologists can evaluate infants in the NICU, pediatric intensive care unit, or in conjunction with other examinations or procedures conducted under general anesthesia or sedation.

Audiological diagnostic evaluation should follow evidence-based protocols and include all aspects of evaluation, not just a single test or

TABLE 10.1

Factors to consider in establishing pediatric audiological diagnostic services

- How many sites can currently perform newborn audiological evaluations?
- How many sites will be needed for the projected birth cohort and projected number of referrals?
- Is there a plan to assure timely diagnosis of children referred from UNHS?
- How far will families need to travel to the diagnostic sites?
- Is teleaudiology a possibility?
- Is adequate equipment available at existing sites to conduct evidence-based audiological diagnostic evaluations of infants?
  - How much equipment will be needed for a sufficient number of diagnostic sites?
  - What is the plan for obtaining equipment?
- Should separate equipment be purchased for each audiological test required?
  - If equipment is multipurpose, what would happen if it needs repair?
- Do existing sites have the equipment required to perform behavioral testing of each ear separately (preferably using insert earphones), by VRA or CPA depending on the developmental age of the child? Speakers in the sound field at 90 degrees azimuth to the right and left are required. ABRs and/or ASSRs, using both air-conduction and bone-conduction transducers, allow the determination of thresholds in children too young or too developmentally immature to test reliably and validly by behavioral methods. OAE equipment is essential to determine cochlear status, tympanometry is essential to determine middle ear status, and otoscopy is required to ensure that the ear canal is patent
- What is the calibration schedule for the equipment?
- Does the facility have the capacity for testing with sedation, if required?
- What is the infection control protocol?
- Is there an evidence-based protocol for the audiological assessment of infants and very young children for the diagnosis of hearing loss and fitting of amplification (if not, a protocol needs to be developed)?

CONTINUED

TABLE 10.1 CONTINUED

- Do personnel have experience of assessing hearing in newborns? Can they:
  - determine the status of the middle ear in newborns and the type of hearing loss (conductive, sensorineural, mixed) without otoscopic examination, because the newborn's ear drums are not likely to be visible?
  - obtain threshold information in both ears sufficient for both diagnosing the hearing loss and fitting amplification in a single session?
  - conduct the appropriate tests to determine ANSD, the status of hearing through neural pathways, and disorders of the eighth auditory nerve?
  - obtain thresholds through VRA and CPA in children 6–30 months of age that are sufficient for fitting amplification devices (at least one high- and one low-frequency threshold in each ear)?
- If personnel lack the experience required, is there a training program that will assure evidence-based practice?
- Who provides the hearing care – audiologists only, ENT physicians only, or both audiologists and ENT physicians?
  - How many audiologists and ENT physicians are in the screening geographic area?
- Will ENT physicians or non-pediatric audiologists need to be trained to conduct diagnostic evaluations of infants?
  - How will training be provided?

ASSR, auditory steady-state response; CPA, conditioned play audiometry; ENT, ear, nose and throat; VRA, visual reinforcement audiometry.

subset of tests. Comprehensive audiological diagnostic evaluation of newborns should aim to gather information about:

- the type of hearing loss (sensorineural, conductive, mixed, auditory neuropathy)
- the degree/severity (frequency-specific thresholds for air- and bone-conduction stimuli) of hearing loss in each ear

- the configuration of the hearing loss in each ear
- the age of onset
- whether the hearing loss is progressive, non-progressive or fluctuating (this will require follow-up)
- whether the hearing loss is unilateral or bilateral
- whether the hearing loss is symmetrical
- the presence or absence of vestibular dysfunction.

Audiological diagnostic evaluation is an ongoing process to determine the stability or progression of the hearing loss, the optimal amplification fit for the thresholds calculated and earmold adjustments, as well as the presence/absence of middle ear involvement.

Case history. The audiological diagnostic evaluation begins with a comprehensive case history to obtain information that may assist in identifying the cause of hearing loss. When referral occurs within the first few weeks of life, a CMV screening test should be conducted to identify cCMV infection, while a referral for genetic screening may identify genes related to hearing loss (see Chapter 5).

Otoscopic examination of newborns may be unrevealing because of difficulties viewing the ear drum, but it can identify the presence of fluid or debris in the ear canal.

Behavioral observation can provide information about any startle response to loud sounds and whether the newborn turns his or her eyes – or even his or her head – toward a sound source. The motor abilities of a newborn will develop with age, allowing more observations. Initially, observations will focus on newborn reflexes and facial expressions.

Infection control policies are vital throughout all stages of audiological evaluation. Their importance has been highlighted particularly during the COVID-19 pandemic and they will continue to be necessary because of the prevalence of viral infections.

Audiological assessment

Infant audiological assessment and determination of hearing thresholds requires not only adherence to best practices, but also sufficient time, space, skill, appropriate equipment and protocols, and patience.

Audiological assessment of infants and young children comprises a number of aspects (Table 10.2). Multiple tests are needed to cross check diagnostic results.[8] The cross-check principle is effective when employing visual reinforcement audiometry (VRA), OAE and tympanometry to rule out or determine the degree, type and configuration of hearing loss in infants.[9,10]

Electrophysiological evaluation. ABR-evoked potentials using click and frequency-specific stimuli are the gold-standard means of determining hearing thresholds in infants under 6 months of age.[4–6,11–20] Because ABR is not a test of hearing, but rather a measure of an electrophysiological response to auditory stimulation, confirmation of hearing (perception) requires behavioral evaluation as soon as the child is developmentally capable of providing reliable and valid behavioral responses to sound.

In the diagnostic ABR, recording the electrophysiological response requires the newborn or infant to sleep soundly for a prolonged period of time so that quiet responses, unmarred by artifact and noise, can be obtained. In the young infant, natural sleep recordings are quite feasible with appropriate preparation. In some cases, sedation or anesthesia is required to ensure sufficient quiet time for all diagnostic measures to be completed.

When possible, it is recommended that middle ear and OAE testing be completed at the beginning of ABR evaluation. This is because some pressure can develop in the middle ear with sedation or deep sleep, which may compromise the middle ear and OAE findings. Frequency-specific (tone-burst/narrow-band chirps) stimuli are used to elicit neural responses that enable determination of thresholds and form the foundation for determining hearing aid amplification characteristics. Tone-burst ABR results at lower frequencies are more likely to overestimate hearing thresholds (suggesting hearing loss when there is none, or resulting in overamplification at low frequencies), while tone-burst threshold estimates at higher

TABLE 10.2

Key aspects of audiological assessment for infants and young children

Electrophysiological evaluation
• ABR is the gold-standard test for threshold estimation for infants and children who cannot complete behavioral audiological assessment • ABR provides ear- and frequency-specific threshold estimation necessary for diagnosis of the type, degree and configuration of hearing loss and provision of amplification[4]
Middle ear evaluation
• Measures of middle ear function should be completed as part of the diagnostic audiological process for infants and young children • Either tympanometry and/or wideband measures can be used to characterize middle ear function[5] • Acoustic reflexes are an important test of middle ear function and the integrity of auditory brainstem pathways[6]
OAE testing
• OAE testing provides important information about the integrity of the outer hair cells in the cochlea and critical information about the differential diagnosis of ANSD and SNHL[1]
Behavioral assessment
• Gold standard for estimation of hearing thresholds • VRA (for infants aged 6–24 months)[2] and CPA (for toddlers aged ≥24 months)[3] are established methods based on conditioned responses to sound

CPA, conditioned play audiometry.

frequencies tend to underestimate hearing thresholds (suggesting that hearing is better than it actually is, or resulting in underamplification at higher frequencies).[13–15]

Auditory steady-state response (ASSR)/chirp thresholds tend to be closer at low frequencies.[16,17]

Thresholds for both air- and bone-conducted stimuli are measured to determine the type (conductive, sensorineural, mixed) of hearing loss. Bone conduction thresholds are necessary for estimating additional hearing aid gain and output if there is a conductive component.

It is theoretically possible that an infant can have normal ABR recordings, yet not be able to perceive or understand the signal, since comprehension occurs at a higher level in the brain than the sites from which an ABR is recorded. When the ABR shows no response, a specialized protocol (around 80 dB normal hearing level click stimulus at positive and negative polarities) should be completed to assess possible auditory neuropathy (see Chapter 13).

Behavioral assessment. Research has indicated a good correlation between average tone, chirp[18–20] and ASSR thresholds and behavioral thresholds at middle to high frequencies in infants and young children. For individual children at individual frequencies, the thresholds may show large discrepancies (±40 dB), necessitating behavioral threshold validation as quickly as possible to assure optimal amplification fit.

Pure-tone thresholds are recognized as the gold standard for determining hearing status.[9,10] VRA is a conditioned response and uses the development of auditory localization in the horizontal plane to observe and reinforce head-turn behavior in response to pure-tone and speech stimuli. Infants are typically able to provide VRA thresholds after 6 months of age. When VRA is conducted according to careful stimulus, response and conditioning protocols, valid and reliable results can be obtained from the typically developing infant.[4–6] Audiometric threshold estimations obtained via VRA are referred to as 'minimum response levels' as they reflect the lowest intensity level at which a response is observed.[4–6]

Assessing infants and young children who cannot be evaluated using behavioral testing. Approximately 40% of young children who are DHH have coexisting conditions that may make audiological evaluation challenging (physical, intellectual, psychological or emotional needs or barriers),[21] requiring specialized training and skills to obtain behavioral results. The benefits and risks must be carefully weighed if older children who cannot be evaluated by behavioral testing are recommended for electrophysiological testing requiring sedation. Medically fragile children may not be candidates for anesthesia.

Middle ear measures. During diagnostic audiological evaluation, measures of middle ear movement assist in the differentiation of conductive and sensory or neural sites. The standard measure for detecting MEF has long been high-frequency tympanometry, because of its superior sensitivity and specificity in detecting MEF or effusion in infants as compared with standard 226 Hz tympanometry. Use of the 1000 Hz probe tone is recommended in infants up to the age of 9 months.[4–6,9,10,22]

Increasingly, wideband acoustic immittance measures are being studied and used in neonates, as these are reported to show superior sensitivity and specificity. CHL can be detected in infants using either 1000 Hz tympanometry or wideband measures.[10,22]

Congenital ossicular abnormalities can be present and can be distinguished by the audiologist using a combination of air- versus bone-conduction threshold estimation in addition to tympanometry, acoustic reflex threshold tests and OAE testing, as well as the otologist's examination and radiographic studies.

Assessing infants/toddlers with middle ear effusion or retained amniotic fluid.[23] Middle ear effusion often complicates the evaluation process, resulting in delayed diagnosis of hearing loss. It is not uncommon for middle ear effusion or retained amniotic fluid in the middle ear to persist in infants regardless of hearing status, causing referral from newborn hearing screening and/or (temporary) CHL (see Chapter 7). The management of MEF should be coordinated by the infant's pediatrician/primary care provider and/or a pediatric otologist, with an audiologist's input, taking the family's preference into account. In some cases, myringotomy with or without placement of a pressure equalization tube will be necessary to complete diagnostic evaluation in a timely fashion during the critical developmental period of early infancy.[24,25]

Acoustic (middle ear muscle) reflex threshold measurement is completed using a 1000 Hz probe tone for newborns and infants under 9 months of age.[4–6] The acoustic reflex can be reliably measured in infants with normal tympanograms and can assist in the diagnosis of peripheral and neural hearing involvement. Good reliability has been shown for tonal and broadband stimuli,[26,27] with published normative data. It is important to recognize that in infants the intensity of the stimulus tone or noise will be greater than the dial setting, as the infant ear canal is considerably smaller than the standard coupler used for calibration.

Normative data for acoustic stapedial reflexes in healthy neonates have shown that reflexes occur at a mean of 57 dB hearing level (db HL) for broadband noise, and range from 65–81 dB HL for tonal stimuli.[26,27] As such, caution must be used in setting the upper limit of stimulus intensity used in eliciting the reflex. The acoustic reflex test is particularly helpful in cases where auditory neuropathy is suspected, as the reflexes are abnormal, most often absent.

Otoacoustic emissions. Diagnostic OAEs provide information about the presence/absence of active cochlear processes, including outer hair cell function, from which hearing level (typical versus elevated) can be inferred, when the middle ear has been shown to be free of effusion. OAE (DPOAE or transient evoked [TEOAE]) testing is essential in pediatric diagnostic evaluation.[28–30] OAEs are measurable sounds that can occur spontaneously or in response to low-intensity stimuli such as clicks and tones. The OAEs are recorded via a probe assembly with a microphone placed in the external ear canal (see Chapter 1). Although it is possible to have OAEs in the presence of mild sensory hearing loss, the magnitude of the emission diminishes with increasingly elevated thresholds, and the emissions are not observed at thresholds greater than 30–35 dB HL.

Mild degrees of hearing loss are difficult to define using OAE technology. The magnitudes of infant OAEs are greater than those of adults, especially at higher frequencies, which facilitates the detection of responses and reduces the impact of low-frequency noise interference. Generally, infants with TEOAEs/DPOAEs are predicted to have hearing thresholds better than 30 dB HL while those with absent TEOAEs/DPOAEs (in the presence of normal tympanometry or wideband measures) are predicted to have hearing thresholds poorer than 30 dB HL.[26–30]

OAE assessment is not sufficient for determining hearing thresholds, and it cannot be used in isolation to determine hearing aid specifications. It is important to remember that OAE only reflects activity in the cochlea. Infants with auditory neuropathy or more central auditory pathologies are expected to have normal OAE, yet clearly do not have normal auditory function.

Future directions

Gathering more information about the prevalence of progressive and acquired hearing loss, as well as mixed hearing loss, in early childhood after newborn hearing screening is important. Increased research in these areas will improve hearing screening for toddlers, preschool- (3–5 years) and school-aged children.[31,32]

Key points – pediatric diagnostic audiology

- Timely, accurate diagnosis of hearing loss is essential for quality EHDI services.
- Audiological diagnosis is optimally carried out by 2–3 months of age when infants are more likely to sleep for prolonged periods, allowing assessment to be carried out without sedation.
- ABR-evoked potentials are the gold-standard means of determining hearing thresholds in infants under 6 months of age but should be confirmed with behavioral testing where possible.
- High-frequency tympanometry has been the standard measure for detecting MEF but wideband measures are increasingly being studied and used with neonates because of their reported superior sensitivity and specificity.
- Acoustic reflexes and ABR are expected to be absent in infants with auditory neuropathy.
- OAE testing reflects activity in the cochlea and is not sufficient for determining hearing thresholds or hearing aid specifications.

References

1. Yoshinaga-Itano C, Sedey AL, Mason CA et al. Early intervention and parent talk predicts pragmatic language in children with hearing loss. *Pediatrics* 2020; 146(suppl 3):S270–7.
2. Yoshinaga-Itano C, Sedey AL, Wiggin M, Mason CA. Language outcomes improved through early hearing detection and earlier cochlear implantation. *Otol Neurotol* 2018;39:1256–63.
3. Yoshinaga-Itano C, Sedey AL, Wiggin M, Chung C. Early hearing detection and vocabulary of children with hearing loss. *Pediatrics* 2017;140:e20162964.
4. Joint Committee on Infant Hearing. Year 2019 position statement: principles and guidelines for early hearing detection and intervention programs. *J Early Hear Detect Interv* 2019;4:1–44.
5. Joint Committee on Infant Hearing. Year 2007 position statement: principles and guidelines for early hearing detection and intervention programs. *Pediatrics* 2007; 120:898–921.
6. Joint Committee on Infant Hearing. Year 2000 position statement: principles and guidelines for early hearing detection and intervention programs. *Pediatrics* 2000; 106:798–817.
7. American Academy of Audiology. Audiologic Guidelines for the Assessment of Hearing in Infants and Young Children, 2012. audiology-web.s3.amazonaws.com/migrated/201208_AudGuideAssessHear_youth.pdf_5399751b249593.36017703.pdf, last accessed 29 June 2021.
8. Norrix LW. Hearing thresholds, minimum response levels, and cross-check measures in pediatric audiology. *Am J Audiol* 2015;24:137–44.
9. Baldwin SM, Gajewski BJ, Widen JE. An evaluation of the cross-check principle using visual reinforcement audiometry, otoacoustic emissions, and tympanometry. *J Am Acad Audiol* 2010;21: 187–96.
10. Prieve BA, Beauchaine KL, Sabo D et al. Evidence-based systematic review of newborn hearing screening using behavioral audiometric threshold as a gold standard. American Speech-Language-Hearing Association, 2013. www.asha.org/siteassets/uploadedFiles/EBSR-Newborn-Hearing-Screening.pdf, last accessed 29 June 2021.
11. Gorga MP, Johnson TA, Kaminski JR et al. Using a combination of click- and tone burst-evoked auditory brain stem response measurements to estimate pure-tone thresholds. *Ear Hear* 2006;2:60–74.

12. Widen JE, Keener SK. Diagnostic testing for hearing loss in infants and young children. *Ment Retard Dev Disabil Res Rev* 2003;9:220–4.
13. Stapells DR, Gravel JS, Martin BA. Thresholds for auditory brain stem responses to tones in notched noise from infants and young children with normal hearing or sensorineural hearing loss. *Ear Hear* 1995;16:361–71.
14. McCreery RW, Kaminski J, Beauchaine K et al. The impact of degree of hearing loss on auditory brainstem response predictions of behavioral thresholds. *Ear Hear* 2015; 36:309–19.
15. Vander Werff KR, Prieve BA, Georgantas LM. Infant air and bone conduction tone burst auditory brain stem responses for classification of hearing loss and the relationship to behavioral thresholds. *Ear Hear* 2009;30:350–68. Erratum in *Ear Hear* 2010;31:379.
16. Rance G, Roper R, Symons L et al. Hearing threshold estimation in infants using auditory steady-state responses. *J Am Acad Audiol* 2005;16: 291–300.
17. Vander Werff KR. Accuracy and time efficiency of two ASSR analysis methods using clinical test protocols. *J Am Acad Audiol* 2009;20:433–52.
18. Xu ZM, Cheng WX, Yao ZH. Prediction of frequency-specific hearing threshold using chirp auditory brainstem response in infants with hearing losses. *Int J Pediatr Otorhinolaryngol* 2014;78:812–16.
19. Cebulla M, Elberling C. Auditory brain stem responses evoked by different chirps based on different delay models. *J Am Acad Audiol* 2015;21:452–60.
20. Cebulla M, Lurz H, Shehata-Dieler W. Evaluation of waveform, latency and amplitude values of chirp ABR in newborns. *Int J Pediatr Otorhinolaryngol* 2014;78:631–6.
21. Gallaudet Research Institute. Regional and national summary report of data from the 2011–12 annual survey of deaf and hard of hearing children and youth. Washington, DC: GRI, Gallaudet University, 2013; research.gallaudet.edu/Demographics/2012_National_Summary.pdf, last accessed 29 June 2021.
22. Hunter LL, Prieve BA, Kei J, Sanford CA. Pediatric applications of wideband acoustic immittance measures. *Ear Hear* 2013;34(suppl 1): 36S–42S.
23. Holte L, Walker E, Oleson J et al. Factors influencing follow-up to newborn hearing screening for infants who are hard of hearing. *Am J Audiol* 2012;21:163–75.

24. Rosenfeld RM, Schwartz SR, Pynnonen MA et al. Clinical practice guideline: tympanostomy tubes in children – executive summary. *Otolaryngol Head Neck Surg* 2013;149:8–16.
25. Boone RT, Bower CM, Martin PF. Failed newborn hearing screens as presentation for otitis media with effusion in the newborn population. *Int J Pediatr Otorhinolaryngol* 2005;69:393–7.
26. de Lyra-Silva KA, Sanches SGG, Neves-Lobo IF et al. Middle ear muscle reflex measurement in neonates: comparison between 1000Hz and 226Hz probe tones. *Int J Pediatr Otorhinolaryngol* 2015;79:1510–15.
27. Kei J. Acoustic stapedial reflexes in healthy neonates: normative data and test-retest reliability. *J Am Acad Audiol* 2012;23:46–56.
28. Gorga MP, Norton SJ, Sininger YS et al. Identification of neonatal hearing impairment: distortion product otoacoustic emissions during the perinatal period. *Ear Hear* 2000;21:400–24.
29. Widen J, Johnson JL, White KR et al. A multisite study to examine the efficacy of the otoacoustic emission/automated auditory brainstem response newborn hearing screening protocol: results of visual reinforcement audiometry. *Am J Audiol* 2005;14:S200–16.
30. Norton SJ, Gorga MP, Widen JE et al. Identification of neonatal hearing impairment: evaluation of transient evoked otoacoustic emission, distortion product otoacoustic emission, and auditory brain stem response test performance. *Ear Hear* 2000;21:508–28.
31. Prieve BA, Schooling T, Venediktov R, Franceschini N. An evidence-based systematic review on the diagnostic accuracy of hearing screening instruments for preschool- and school-age children. *Am J Audiol* 2015;24:250–67.
32. American Academy of Audiology Subcommittee. American Academy of Audiology Childhood Hearing Screening Guidelines, 2011. www.cdc.gov/ncbddd/hearingloss/documents/aaa_childhood-hearing-guidelines_2011.pdf, last accessed 29 June 2021.

Further reading and resources

American Academy of Audiology. Clinical guidance document. Assessment of hearing in infants and young children, 2020. audiology.org/wp-content/uploads/2021/05/Clin-Guid-Doc_Assess_Hear_Infants_Children_1.23.20-1 last accessed 2 July 2021.

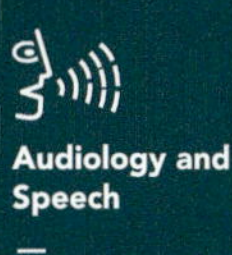

—

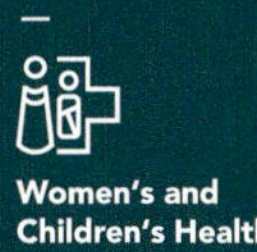

11 Amplification device fitting

Kristin Uhler and Christine Yoshinaga-Itano

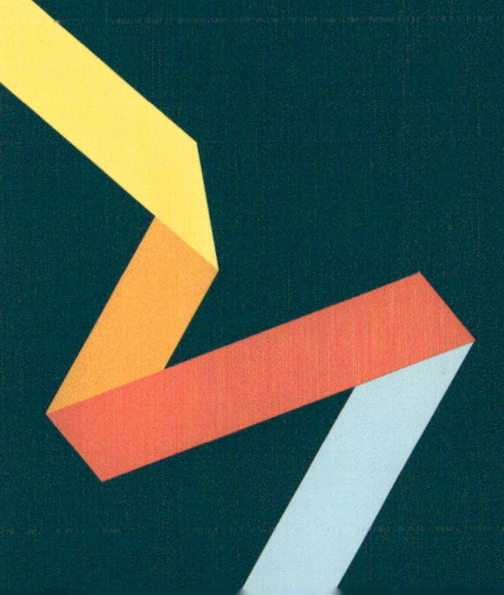

HEALTHCARE

An important first intervention following a diagnosis of hearing loss is the fitting of amplification technology.[1–8] Amplification technology can assist almost all infants and young children with hearing loss but the availability of hearing aid and cochlear implant technology varies across the world and may be dependent on government financial support, personal insurance or on an individual's ability to pay.

Even when hearing aid and cochlear implant technologies are available, evidence-based practice for fitting amplification is not uniform, even in high-income countries.[9] If the technology is not properly fitted, infants and young children may not have access to all of the sounds of their native language necessary for them to develop speech.

Amplification in infants and young children

No child is too young to be a candidate for amplification,[1–3] nor does an auditory evoked potential (AEP) result of 'no response' exclude a child from being fitted with amplification. Children with bilateral and unilateral SNHL (even when it is minimal), permanent CHL, ANSD or CHL that is unresolved after 6 months of treatment should be considered for amplification.

For infants or children with peripheral hearing loss, the decision to use amplification technology will be made by their parents, with input from an audiologist and, ideally, from a parent-to-parent support or peer support source.[1–3] If parents set a goal of achieving oral/spoken language, audiological counseling regarding the importance of hearing aid and/or cochlear implant amplification is necessary. If the child has significant profound hearing loss and parents desire oral/ spoken language, cochlear implants may be the only intervention that can provide the infant with access to spoken language.

Programs should strive to provide amplification for a child within 1 month of the diagnosis of hearing loss and to fit amplification by 2–3 months of age. The goal is to meet the EHDI 1–3–6 benchmarks and, if possible, EHDI 1–2–3 (see Chapter 1). Earlier amplification following diagnosis has been shown to significantly affect the development of communication outcomes in terms of auditory skills (listening) and understanding and producing spoken language.[10–13]

Hearing aids

Hearing aid fitting proceeds optimally when the results of physiological and audiological assessment, including diagnostic AEP,

OAE, tympanometry and medical examination, show agreement. For infants younger than 6 months of age, hearing aid selection will be based on physiological measures alone. Tone-burst/chirp AEP thresholds will be used for initial hearing aid fitting, but as soon as developmentally possible, behavioral threshold assessment using VRA is essential to cross-check and augment physiological findings and verify hearing aid gain and output targets.[14]

Bilateral amplification is recommended unless there are medical or audiological contraindications, such as significantly poorer discrimination in one ear, issues with sound crossing over to the better ear and/or creating a distorted signal, absence/malformation of a cochlear or auditory nerve, or chronic middle ear involvement in one ear. The choice of sound transmission (air versus bone conduction) is based on the type and severity of the hearing loss and physical features of the outer ear, with osseointegrated devices (BAHAs) designed for children with CHL and unilateral deafness (Table 11.1).[2]

TABLE 11.1

Hearing aid considerations for children with UHL and/or CHL

- In children younger than 5 years, a bone conduction signal can be transmitted via a non-surgical bone conduction hearing device attached to the child using a headband, softband, adhesive, eyeglasses or another mechanism[15]
- In children aged 5 years and older, surgically implanted bone-anchored hearing implants can be used[15]
- Use of a bone conduction signal may be an effective means of amplification for children with bilateral CHL
- Use of a bone conduction signal may be an option for children with UHL
  - For children with single-sided deafness, a cochlear implant should be considered; countries differ on candidacy approval and in the USA the Food and Drug Administration has approved implantation for children older than 5 years with single-sided deafness
- As children become more active, FM/DM systems with a wireless remote microphone receiver may be considered. Infants and young children may benefit from FM/DM technology particularly in noisy situations, such as in automobiles, restaurants, outdoors or in groups of children

FM/DM, frequency modulation/digital modulation.

Bimodal sound transmission – a cochlear implant in one ear and a hearing aid on the other – is recommended for children with unilateral cochlear implants and for infants learning tonal language in the home, depending on the amount of residual hearing.[1–5]

Choice of hearing aid should include consideration of:[1–4]

- gain and output requirements
- frequency bandwidth
- ear canal size and shape
- expected changes in concha and ear canal size
- occlusion
- skin sensitivity
- need for specific features such as a directional microphone, telecoil, direct auditory input, built-in frequency modulation/digital modulation (FM/DM) receiver or reserve gain
- selection options including (but not limited to) pediatric features such as style, color, retention devices, pediatric ear hooks and filters for analog aids
- childproofing measures such as tamperproof battery doors
- parental choice regarding device esthetics

Behind-the-ear (BTE) hearing aids are the style of choice while a child is growing and provide the features required for pediatric patients. Standard BTE hearing aids should provide appropriate coupling with assistive devices. Some manufacturers offer trials of different hearing aids and loaner hearing aid programs.

Tubing size, occlusion and receiver placement are individual choices based on patient communication needs and preferences, ear canal dimensions, and hearing loss severity and configuration. However, receiver-in-the-canal or mini BTE hearing aids should not be fitted on infants.

Verification, optimization and validation. Hearing aids for infants and children must be fitted and optimized individually based on the real ear-to-coupler difference (RECD).[14] Using a manufacturer's proprietary 'first-fit' algorithms in the absence of real ear verification is not appropriate. RECD is also preferred to the use of age-average measures.

An evidence-based target prescription (such as the Desired Sensation Level or the National Acoustic Laboratories prescriptive methods)[7,14,16,17] should be used when fitting and verifying hearing aids. The aided speech intelligibility index (SII) has been shown to be a strong predictor of spoken language development and should be reported for each hearing aid fitting, preferably aiming for an SII of 0.70 or greater.[7]

Verification and optimization should be repeated each time a new earmold is fitted, when there are changes in hearing thresholds and also on long-term validation. Infants and young children should have their hearing sensitivity/thresholds examined every 3 months for the first 3 years of life, then every 6 months until they enter school and then at least annually thereafter. Ongoing validation, with assessment of speech discrimination (Table 11.2),[18,19] is mandatory to ensure that the purpose of hearing aids – facilitating access to spoken language – is being maximized by the child's amplification and/or prosthetic devices.

Earmolds. Because the ear canal grows rapidly during early childhood, it is vital that earmolds are replaced at least every 3 months in infancy and every year after the first year of life. Be proactive about earmold replacement; commonly, when a child changes a shoe size, they will need a new earmold (Table 11.3).

Cochlear implantation

Cochlear implantation at younger ages is related to better developmental and language outcomes,[20] and new research and technological advancements mean that pediatric cochlear implantation candidacy is rapidly evolving.[21–23] The criteria for candidacy in children are ever-changing and physicians should

TABLE 11.2

Validation of hearing aid fitting

- Validation of infant hearing aid fitting can be accomplished after 6–7 months of age through visual reinforcement of infant speech discrimination,[18,19] a technique similar to VRA using speech phoneme discrimination
- In older children validation of hearing aid fitting is accomplished through speech recognition testing

TABLE 11.3

Tips for earmold making and use in infants and young children

- Use a soft earmold material
- Provide a long canal length to prevent an occlusion effect
- Guard against reverse horns created by crimping the end of the sound channel in small earmolds
- Approach venting cautiously in pediatric earmolds because of space limitations and the additional challenge of feedback
- Use pediatric ear hooks to promote retention
- Use filtered ear hooks to promote a smooth frequency response
- Use automatic feedback suppression with caution; if feedback requires gain to be decreased and the child's hearing aids no longer meet the prescriptive gain targets then new earmolds should be made

always refer to the current rules applicable in their own countries. Some candidacy recommendations have gained approval from country-specific entities (for example, the Australian Therapeutic Goods Administration, Belgian Federal Government, British Cochlear Implant Group, Danish National Board of Health, European 'CE' marking and US Food and Drug Administration [FDA]), whereas others reflect guidelines from individual cochlear implant manufacturers or evidence-based practice that is used before official changes are made to approved guidelines.[24–26]

Most guidelines worldwide agree on the validity of pediatric implantation for profound bilateral hearing loss, but differences arise in the age at implantation, the level of residual hearing, speech recognition and auditory status of the contralateral ear.[27–29] While children of younger ages receive implantation in the USA, Europe and Australia, there is limited evidence of any advantage being gained from children receiving implantation younger than age 9–12 months.

In the USA, children of 9–18 months of age are eligible for cochlear implantation if they have profound SNHL of 90 dB or greater in both ears, while children of 24 months of age or older become eligible if they have severe-to-profound SNHL of 70 dB or greater in both ears.

The FDA has recently also approved the use of specific devices for individuals with single-sided deafness, or asymmetric SNHL. However, great variance exists in protocols for candidacy determination for children across cochlear implantation centers in the USA.

Bilateral cochlear implantation has been shown to result in significant benefits over unilateral implantation, particularly in the ability to localize sound sources. As previously mentioned, bimodal cochlear implantation, with a hearing aid on the other ear, may be appropriate for children learning tonal languages.[30]

Hearing aid trial. In general, it is recommended that, unless there is a medical contraindication, a child is appropriately fitted with hearing aids and uses them for 3–6 months before determining whether they are candidates for cochlear implantation. In cases of meningitis, a younger age at implantation and a shorter hearing aid trial is recommended; the trial may be waived in some cases as bony growth in the cochlea following meningitis may interfere with or complicate cochlear implantation.

Children who gain limited benefit from conventional amplification (Table 11.4) are considered candidates for cochlear implantation if they have poor speech perception, unaided pure-tone thresholds greater than 70 dB, poor functional performance, limited language progress or auditory development, or poor quality of life.[31–37]

Timing of implantation. Children with progressive hearing loss should be assessed for cochlear implantation as soon as they become eligible based on the degree of hearing loss. There are advantages to

TABLE 11.4

Evidence of lack of benefit from appropriately set hearing aids

- Inconsistent response to his/her name in quiet environment with amplification
- Failure to alert to environmental sounds while wearing amplification
- Failure to identify/repeat back the LIng 6 sounds ('ah', 'ee', 'oo', 's', 'sh', 'm') or the sound equivalents in the child's native language

sequential implants, particularly when residual low-frequency hearing exists in the non-implanted ear, which can be amplified through a well-fitted hearing aid to maximize low-frequency speech cues.

Contraindications may prevent or delay implantation or may alter expectations for long-term outcomes (Table 11.5). Other barriers to early cochlear implantation include delays in insurance approval, family indecision and geographic location.[38]

Counseling. Parents of infants and children who are candidates for cochlear implantation will want to learn more about it, and physicians should share information with them at all stages of the process. Parents must have realistic expectations and should be advised of the advantages and limitations of the technology and made aware that cochlear implantation is a powerful tool to enable access to spoken language development in deaf children but is not a cure for deafness.

TABLE 11.5

Contraindications to cochlear implantation

- Absent or abnormal auditory nerve, absent/malformed cochlea
  - Implanting children with an auditory nerve deficiency may result in poorer outcomes. Auditory nerve deficiency can range from relatively minor to complete; imaging with MRI and CT provides optimal assessment of the status of the auditory nerve
- Medical conditions or developmental delays that would severely limit participation in aural habilitation, although significant improvements in quality of life have been demonstrated for individuals with severe-to-profound neurological injuries, cognitive challenges and/or autism
- ANSD with good speech recognition irrespective of degree of hearing loss
- Active middle ear infections

Educational and home environment. All families with the goal of developing listening and spoken language should be in a rehabilitative (home or clinic) or educational setting that emphasizes the development of auditory (listening and spoken language) skills. Families must be committed to using amplification technology as well as exposing children to quality listening and spoken language experiences. Rehabilitative or educational environments that encourage auditory skill development have a positive effect on the child's listening and spoken language progress.

Children with auditory neuropathy spectrum disorder

Either hearing aids or cochlear implantation may support good outcomes in children with ANSD depending on the site of the lesion in the auditory system. It is important to judge each child individually to determine whether implantation or hearing aid(s) or bimodal stimulation is the best option. When a child with ANSD shows no response on the ABR diagnostic evaluation, it is imperative to not solely rely on the degree of hearing loss, but also consider the child's speech recognition abilities, both with and without hearing aids.

Cortical AEPs can provide useful information about the best approach to treatment in children with ANSD. Cortical AEPs are present in two-thirds of children with ANSD, while the remaining one-third will have absent or abnormal responses.[39] ASSR thresholds can also be valuable objective measures of hearing thresholds and have been found to be detectable in 73% of children with ANSD.[40]

Providing quality care

Hospital/state/provincial/national programs that provide amplification to infants and young children identified with hearing loss through UNHS should evaluate their ability to provide an evidence-based quality program. Both programmatic and personnel needs must be addressed (Table 11.6).

TABLE 11.6

Programmatic and personnel considerations in providing amplification services

Financial and equipment readiness

- How will sufficient funding be obtained to train personnel and purchase the amplification devices, programming and verification equipment, and software needed to fit infants identified with hearing loss as soon as possible after identification?
- Does the amplification device fitting facility have the following?
  - Real ear measurement and electroacoustic analysis equipment to measure the output of a hearing aid in an infant's/child's ear canal and assess hearing aid function
  - Hearing aid analyzer to assess hearing aid function compared with manufacturer specifications
  - Earmold facility
  - Batteries
- Can the facility assure daily calibration of equipment by an audiologist/hearing specialist and annual calibration and preventative maintenance by individuals who adhere to American National Standards Institute, International Organization for Standardization and International Electrotechnical Commission standards?
- What provisions/financial support will be available for families unable to purchase amplification, batteries, earmolds and replacements?
- Which fitting protocol for pediatric amplification will be used?
- Is a computer available, with necessary software and internet capacity, to program hearing aids and cochlear implants?

Personnel and training readiness

- Can the facility assure that professionals who determine candidacy and fit amplification are well trained and follow evidence-based practice protocols?
- What training is provided to staff assessing infants with hearing loss, fitting amplification and programming cochlear implants?
- Is training provided to staff on:
  - candidacy, preselection issues and procedures
  - digital signal processing

CONTINUED

TABLE 11.6 CONTINUED

Personnel and training readiness (*cont'd*)

- – hearing instrument selection/fitting considerations
- – fitting verification
- – hearing instrument orientation and training
- – fitting validation, follow-up and referral
- What are the necessary staff competencies related to amplification (hearing aid) fitting? Who will undertake precochlear implant evaluation when appropriate?
- If training is needed, how will that be provided?

Key points – amplification device fitting

- No child is too young to be a candidate for amplification and early amplification is associated with better communication outcomes.
- BTE hearing aids are the style of choice in growing children, with bilateral amplification generally recommended.
- Hearing aids must be fitted and optimized for every child individually using the RECD difference measure.
- Earmolds require regular replacement as a child grows.
- Pediatric cochlear implantation is a valid option for profound hearing loss, but the criteria for candidacy vary from country to country and change frequently.
- A 3–6-month trial of hearing aid amplification should be undertaken before assessing a child for cochlear implantation.
- Parents of children who are candidates for implantation should have realistic expectations of the technology.
- The use of amplification technology and exposure of the child to listening and spoken language experiences should be encouraged in family environments where the goal is for the child to develop listening and spoken language.
- Children with ANSD can benefit from hearing aids or cochlear implants depending on the lesion location in their auditory system.

References

1. Joint Committee on Infant Hearing. Year 2000 position statement: principles and guidelines for early hearing detection and intervention programs. *Pediatrics* 2000; 106:798–817.
2. Joint Committee on Infant Hearing. Year 2007 position statement: principles and guidelines for early hearing detection and intervention programs. *Pediatrics* 2007; 120:898–921.
3. Joint Committee on Infant Hearing. Year 2019 position statement: principles and guidelines for early hearing detection and intervention programs. *J Early Hear Detect Interv* 2019;4:1–44.
4. American Academy of Audiology. Clinical Practice Guidelines on Pediatric Amplification. Reston, VA: American Academy of Audiology, 2013. http://audiology-web.s3.amazonaws.com/migrated/PediatricAmplificationGuidelines.pdf_539975b3e7e9f1.74471798.pdf, last accessed 20 July 2021.
5. Bagatto M, Scollie SD, Hyde M, Seewald R. Protocol for the provision of amplification within the Ontario infant hearing program. *Int J Audiol* 2010;49(suppl 1):S70–9.
6. Bagatto M, Moodie S, Scollie S et al. Clinical protocols for hearing instrument fitting in the Desired Sensation Level method. *Trends Amplif* 2005;9:199–226.
7. Ching TY, Johnson EE, Hou S et al. A comparison of NAL and DSL prescriptive methods for paediatric hearing-aid fitting: predicted speech intelligibility and loudness. *Int J Audiol* 2013;52(suppl 2):S29–38.
8. Orji A, Kamenov,K, Dirac M et al. Global and regional needs, unmet needs and access to hearing aids. *Int J Audiol* 2020;59:166–172.
9. McCreery RW, Bentler RA, Roush PA. Characteristics of hearing aid fittings in infants and young children. *Ear Hear* 2013;34:701–10.
10. McCreery RW, Walker EA, Stiles DJ et al. Audibility-based hearing aid fitting criteria for children with mild bilateral hearing loss. *Lang Speech Hear Serv Sch* 2020;51:55–67.
11. McCreery RW, Walker EA, Spratford M et al. Longitudinal predictors of aided speech audibility in infants and children. *Ear Hear* 2015; 36(suppl 1):S24–37.
12. Ching TYC, Dillon H, Button L et al. Age at intervention for permanent hearing loss and 5-year language outcomes. *Pediatrics* 2017;140:e20164274.
13. Sininger YS, Grimes A, Christensen E. Auditory development in early amplified children: factors influencing auditory-based communication outcomes in children with hearing loss. *Ear Hear* 2010; 31:166–85.

14. Bagatto M, Moodie S, Brown C et al. Prescribing and verifying hearing aids applying the American Academy of Audiology Pediatric Amplification Guideline: protocols and outcomes from the Ontario Infant Hearing Program. *J Am Acad Audiol* 2016;27:188–203.
15. Ellsperman SE, Nairn EM, Stucken EZ. Review of bone conduction hearing devices. *Audiol Res* 2021;11:207–19.
16. Moodie STF, Network of Pediatric Audiologists of Canada, Scollie SD et al. Fit-to-targets for the desired sensation level version 5.0a hearing aid prescription method for children. *Am J Audiol* 2017;26:251–8.
17. Scollie S, Levy C, Pourmand N et al. Fitting noise management signal processing applying the American Academy of Audiology Pediatric Amplification Guideline: verification protocols. *J Am Acad Audiol* 2016;27:237–51.
18. Uhler KM, Baca R, Dudas E, Fredrickson T. Refining stimulus parameters in assessing infant speech perception using visual reinforcement infant speech discrimination: sensation level. *J Am Acad Audiol* 2015;26: 807–14.
19. Uhler K, Warner-Czyz A, Gifford R. Pediatric minimum speech test battery. *J Am Acad Audiol* 2017;28:232–47.
20. Uhler K, Yoshinaga-Itano C, Gabbard SA et al. Longitudinal infant speech perception in young cochlear implant users. *J Am Acad Audiol* 2011;22:129–42.
21. Uhler K, Gifford RH. Current trends in pediatric cochlear implant candidate selection and postoperative follow-up. *Am J Audiol* 2014;23:309–25.
22. Leigh JR, Dettman SJ, Dowell RC. Evidence-based guidelines for recommending cochlear implantation for young children: audiological criteria and optimizing age at implantation. *Int J Audiol* 2016;55(suppl 2):S9–18.
23. Varadarajan VV, Sydlowski SA, Li MM et al. Evolving criteria for adult and pediatric cochlear implantation. *Ear Nose Throat J* 2021;100:31–7.
24. American Academy of Audiology. Clinical Practice Guideline: Cochlear Implants. Reston, VA: American Academy of Audiology, 2019. https://apps.asha.org/EvidenceMaps/Articles/ArticleSummary/f54bd21f-91a5-4764-8ec4-2fc67456fd93, last accessed 10 June 2022.
25. Messersmith JJ, Entwisle L, Warren S, Scott M. Clinical practice guidelines: cochlear implants. *J Am Acad Audiol* 2019;30:827–44.
26. British Cochlear Implant Group. Quality Standards Cochlear Implant Services for Children and Adults, 2018. www.bcig.org.uk/wp-content/uploads/2018/05/QS-update-2018-PDF-final.pdf, last accessed 20 July 2021.

27. Vickers D, De Raeve L, Graham J. International survey of cochlear implant candidacy. *Cochlear Implants Int* 2016;17(suppl 1):36–41.
28. Bruijnzeel H, Bezdjian A, Lesinski-Schiedat A et al. Evaluation of pediatric cochlear implant care throughout Europe: is European pediatric cochlear implant care performed according to guidelines? *Cochlear Implants Int* 2017;18:287–96.
29. National Institute for Health and Care Excellence. Cochlear implants for children and adults with severe to profound deafness. Technology Appraisal Guidance [TA566], 2019. www.nice.org.uk/guidance/TA566, last accessed 23 July 2021.
30. Liu Y-W, Tao D-D, Chen B et al. Factors affecting bimodal benefit in pediatric mandarin-speaking chinese cochlear implant users. *Ear Hear* 2019; 40:1316–27.
31. Bittencourt AG, Ikari LS, Della Torre AA et al. Post-lingual deafness: benefits of cochlear implants vs. conventional hearing aids. *Braz J Otorhinolaryngol* 2012;78:124–7.
32. Dettman SJ, D'Costa WA, Dowell RC et al. Cochlear implants for children with significant residual hearing. *Arch Otolaryngol Head Neck Surg* 2004;130:612–8.
33. Davidson LS. Effects of stimulus level on the speech perception abilities of children using cochlear implants or digital hearing aids. *Ear Hear* 2006;27:493–507.
34. Fitzpatrick E, Olds J, Durieux-Smith A, McCrae R et al. Pediatric cochlear implantation: how much hearing is too much? *Int J Audiol* 2009;48:91–7.
35. Leal C, Marriage J, Vickers D. Evaluating recommended audiometric changes to candidacy using the speech intelligibility index. *Cochlear Implants Int* 2016;17(suppl 1): 8–12.
36. Leigh J, Dettman S, Dowell R, Sarant J. Evidence-based approach for making cochlear implant recommendations for infants with residual hearing. *Ear Hear* 2011;32:313–22.
37. Leigh JR, Moran M, Hollow R, Dowell RC. Evidence-based guidelines for recommending cochlear implantation for postlingually deafened adults. *Int J Audiol* 2016;55(suppl 2): S3–8.
38. Armstrong M, Maresh A, Buxton C et al. Barriers to early pediatric cochlear implantation. *Int J Pediatr Otorhinolaryngol* 2013;77:1869–72.
39. Sharma A, Cardon G. Cortical development and neuroplasticity in auditory neuropathy spectrum disorder. *Hear Res* 2015;330:221–32.
40. Lalayants, MR, Brashkina NB, Geptner EN et al. [Auditory evoked potentials in children with auditory neuropathy spectrum disorder.] *Vestn Otorinolaringol* 2018;83:15–20. (in Russian)

Further reading and resources

Advanced Bionics. Are cochlear implants right for your child? https://advancedbionics.com/us/en/home/about-cochlear-implants/the-journey-for-your-child/is-your-child-a-candidate-.html

BabyHearing.org. Cochlear implant candidacy: criteria for cochlear implantation in children. www.babyhearing.org/devices/cochlear-implant-candidacy

BabyHearing.org. Amplification, implants and FM systems for infants and young children with hearing loss. www.babyhearing.org/professional-resources/Documents/AmplificationImplant Technology.pdf

Centers for Disease Control and Prevention. Technology and audiology. www.cdc.gov/ncbddd/hearingloss/parentsguide/hearingloss/intervention-tech.html

Cochlear. Cochlear implant candidacy information. www.cochlear.com/us/en/professionals/products-and-candidacy/candidacy/cochlear-implant

Hands & Voices. Communication considerations: cochlear implants. www.handsandvoices.org/comcon/articles/cochlearimplants.htm

McCreery RW. Automatic hearing aid features and children. Stop and verify. *Hearing J* 2014;67:22–3.

MED-EL. Hearing implants for children. https://s3.medel.com/pdf/21567E_r60_ParentsGuide_web.pdf

National Center for Hearing Assessment and Management, Utah State University. Cochlear implants: determining candidacy for young children. www.infanthearing.org/ehdi-ebook/2017_ebook/11%20Chapter%2011CochlearImplants DeterminingCandidacy2017.pdf

National Institute on Deafness and Other Communication Disorders. Cochlear implants. www.nidcd.nih.gov/health/cochlear-implants

Phonak. Hearing solutions for infants and toddlers. www.phonak.com/us/en/hearing-aids/hearing-aids-for-children/hearing-aids-for-toddlers.html

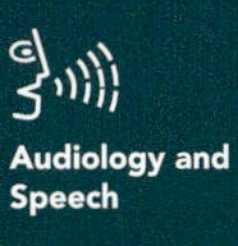

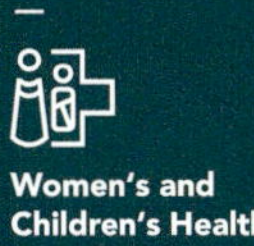

12 Family-centered early intervention

Trudy Smith, Bianca Birdsey, Gwen Carr, Elaine Gale, Christine Yoshinaga-Itano and Daniel Holzinger

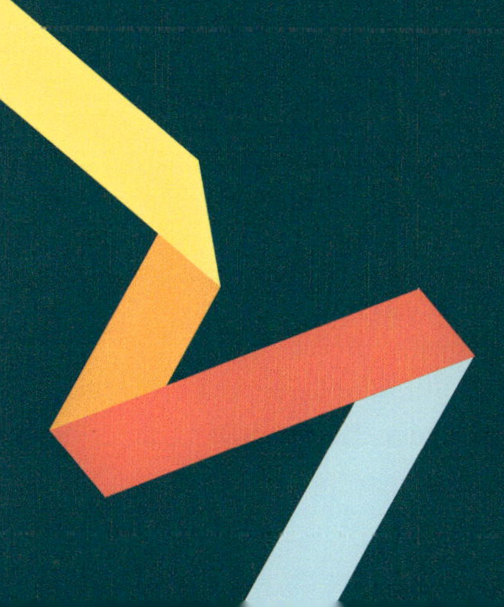

HEALTHCARE

The right to effective language and communication is enshrined in Article 19 of the United Nations *Universal Declaration of Human Rights*.[1] Furthermore, the United Nations *Convention on the Rights of the Child*[2] recognizes the right of every child to 'the highest attainable standard of health', to the development of 'mental and physical abilities to their fullest potential', to optimum socioemotional development and to the opportunity to contribute fully to society. There is now incontrovertible evidence to show that early identification coupled with high-quality diagnostics and intervention can radically improve outcomes in these and other areas for DHH children.

Traditional guidance typically refers to three components that need to be included in an EHDI program.

- Early screening and confirmation that a child is DHH as part of a newborn hearing screening program or as soon after birth as feasible.
- Provision of optimal amplification, such as hearing aids or cochlear implants.
- Engagement in an early intervention program.

Early intervention, however, is too often conceptualized as primarily the provision of amplification devices, with or without some therapeutic professional input for the development of spoken language. FCEI challenges this notion, emphasizing the need for recognition of different approaches to developing language and communication, whether spoken or signed. FCEI is important to support the wellbeing of families and their DHH children, and facilitates the development of effective early intervention programs in which families themselves, and those with the lived experience of being DHH, are involved not only in evaluating the services they receive but also in their design and strategic development.

Family involvement

There is general agreement that providing an EHDI program is crucial to optimizing child outcomes, and that family engagement with early intervention is a key factor. Research shows that 'the single most effective predictor of a newly identified child's success is achieved when early identification is paired with interventions that actively involve families'.[3] The Global Coalition of Parents of Children who are Deaf or Hard of Hearing[4] further calls for EHDI services to recognize that a successful DHH child 'is the product of a well-adjusted, successfully supported family' and that families have different configurations, cultures, 'cultures within cultures', beliefs, values and personal resources. FCEI respects these diversities, recognizing the need to have equal partnerships between families and service providers/mentors, both hearing and DHH, to ensure the optimal development of language and communication skills, and socioemotional and educational development of children who are DHH, through shared goal setting and collaborative relationships at all levels of an EHDI program. There is growing evidence of the influence that engagement in an FCEI program can have on long-term impacts for the child and family.[5–7]

Early communication. Families with children who are DHH face many decisions, both early on and throughout their parenting and life journeys. Many of these decisions are complex and require nuanced understanding of developmental needs, language acquisition, technical details and contextual circumstances.[8]

A major determining factor in the success of a child who is DHH is the meaningful engagement of their family in promoting early communication.[9–14] When a child is identified as DHH, it can disrupt a family's efforts to communicate with the child, leading to a risk of language deprivation or delays in language development and learning, negatively impacting the creation of family bonds (and potentially compromising child safety leading to safeguarding concerns), as well as affecting both socioemotional and cognitive development. The decisions families make for their children at this crucial time are therefore inestimably important.

An effective FCEI program provides balanced information and support to help families understand the risks, benefits and consequences of their potential decisions and to make positive informed choices for their children and themselves. FCEI supports families not only to become competent in their own use of, and encouraging of their child's acceptance of, amplification technology, but also to understand the wider aspects of different approaches to language and communication development, whether visual or oral, engaging them in early communication with their child through the provision of accessible and well-adapted language input.

Peers and mentors. Effective FCEI requires not only professional service provision but also the building of support systems for families in which the lived experience of being DHH can be shared. This can be achieved through family peer support and the involvement of adults who are DHH. Families gain significant support in coping with the confirmation that a child is DHH, as well as knowledge and information, from others who share similar life experiences, increasing their confidence in parenting their DHH child.[15]

In addition to parent/family peers, access to professionals and mentors who are DHH and who have diverse expertise and occupations can be particularly beneficial to families.[16,17] Most families with infants identified through EHDI programs have never known an individual who was born DHH, either child or adult. The ability to interact with adults who are DHH, communicating through signed and/or spoken language, affords families insights into possible futures for their own children, deepening their understanding and enhancing their abilities to support their children to have full access to language and communication, healthy socioemotional development and strong senses of identity.

Factors affecting outcomes

A large body of research has demonstrated the effectiveness of early intervention on the language and learning outcomes of children who are DHH but it is still unknown which elements have the most impact. There is also some conjecture about the effects of different doses and durations of early intervention. Children who are DHH and their families have highly heterogeneous needs, and multiple factors contribute to individual child and family outcomes. Many large-scale studies[5,18–20] have shown that outcomes of family-centered programs are commonly affected by variations in child, family and societal factors, including:

- access to language
- child cognitive abilities
- etiologies
- presence of disabilities
- socioeconomic factors
- educational levels
- societal/cultural norms

- access to quality interventions
- access to technology.[21]

Accessible language environments. A common misconception among medical professionals is that early identification and the provision of amplification devices at a young age will ensure optimal outcomes for children who are DHH. However, access to speech and environmental sounds does not in itself result in access to language and communication competence for a child. A further misconception relates to communication modalities and the perceived superiority of listening and spoken language over manual (signed) languages. Consistent access to language input is essential for all children, including those learning multiple languages. For children who are DHH, accessible language environments that provide consistent communication input that is rich in quality and quantity are particularly important, whether language is signed, spoken, or a combination of signed and spoken. The quality and quantity of direct exposure that children receive to the language(s) around them, the extent to which they can access that language input and the quality of family–child interaction all influence learning and cognition throughout development[11,22–26]

Promoting positive outcomes

The international consensus statement on best practices in FCEI[27] describes ten evidence-informed principles that contribute to positive outcomes (Table 12.1). The principles, which are currently being updated to reflect the latest evidence and leadership from families and providers within early intervention for children who are DHH, promote essential thinking beyond confirmation that a child is DHH and the fitting of amplification technology to build partnerships between families and qualified professionals and to create the optimal circumstances for family wellbeing in which children's development will thrive.

Supportive relationships within the family system and within the community help children and families develop the capacities needed to do well. The Center on the Developing Child at Harvard University emphasizes the value of families gaining knowledge from communities that can provide the 'expertise, wisdom, goals and

TABLE 12.1

Principles underpinning positive outcomes for children who are DHH

- Early, timely and equitable provision of early intervention following identification
- Family–provider partnerships
- Informed choice and decision-making
- Family social and emotional support
- Family–infant interaction
- Use of assistive technologies and supporting means of communication
- Qualified professionals
- Collaborative teamwork
- Progress monitoring
- Program monitoring

values of local leaders and parents who understand what resources and supports are needed'.[22] In this respect, families value and benefit from opportunities to interact with other parents as well as individuals who are DHH.[28–32]

Building an effective FCEI program involves embracing collaborative teamwork as an essential component of achieving differentiation in services for all children who are DHH, including those with special needs. Depending on the needs of the individual child and family, these multidisciplinary teams necessarily include combinations of parents/caregivers, early intervention providers with specialized knowledge and skills in early childhood and early language acquisition, providers with knowledge and skills in working with families of children who are DHH (such as teachers of children who are DHH and speech-language pathologists), otolaryngologists, audiologists, service coordinators, individuals who are DHH (as role models/mentors or in other professional capacities), sign language tutors, social workers and psychologists, and representatives of parent-to-parent support networks.

Key points – family-centered early intervention

- Family-to-family support is a critical component of FCEI services.
- Engaging in an FCEI program can help families make informed decisions and choices to support their child's language development and bring positive long-term benefits to both families and children who are DHH.
- Family involvement in promoting early communication is a major factor in determining the success of a child who is DHH.
- Consistent access to language input, whether signed, spoken or both, is particularly important for children who are DHH.
- The involvement of professionals who are DHH and mentors in FCEI programs gives families insight into what might be possible for their child.
- Effective FCEI programs require collaborative teamwork between families and combinations of professionals and EHDI service providers.

References

1. United Nations. Universal Declaration of Human Rights. www.un.org/en/about-us/universal-declaration-of-human-rights, last accessed 2 July 2021.
2. United Nations. Convention on the Rights of the Child. www.ohchr.org/en/professionalinterest/pages/crc.aspx, last accessed 2 July 2021.
3. Yoshinaga-Itano C. Successful outcomes for deaf and hard of hearing children. *Semin Hearing* 2000;21:309–26.
4. Global Coalition of Parents of Children who are Deaf or Hard of Hearing. Position Statement 2010. www.gpodhh.org/position-statement-2010, last accessed 2 July 2021.
5. Yoshinaga-Itano C, Sedey AL, Wiggin M, Chung C. Early hearing detection and vocabulary of children with hearing loss. *Pediatrics* 2017;140:e20162964.
6. Holzinger D, Fellinger J, Beitel C. Early onset of family centred intervention predicts language outcomes in children with hearing loss. *Int J Pediatr Otorhinolaryngol* 2011;75:256–60.
7. Neumann K, Gross M, Bottcher P et al. Effectiveness and efficiency of a universal newborn hearing screening in Germany. *Folia Phoniatr Logop* 2006;58:440–55.

8. Porter A, Creed P, Hood M, Ching TYC. Parental decision-making and deaf children: a systematic literature review. *J Deaf Stud Deaf Educ* 2018;23:295–306.
9. Cruz I, Quittner AL, Marker C et al. Identification of effective strategies to promote language in deaf children with cochlear implants. *Child Dev* 2013;84:543–59.
10. DesJardin JL, Eisenberg LS. Maternal contributions: supporting language development in young children with cochlear implants. *Ear Hear* 2007; 28:456–69.
11. Holzinger D, Dall M, Sanduvete-Chaves S et al. The impact of family environment on language development of children with cochlear implants: a systematic review and meta-analysis. *Ear Hear* 2020;41:1077–91.
12. Nittrouer S, Lowenstein JH, Antonelli J. Parental language input to children with hearing loss: does it matter in the end? *J Speech Lang Hear Res* 2019;63:234–58.
13. Szagun G, Stumper B. Age or experience? The influence of age at implantation, social and linguistic environment on language development in children with cochlear implants. *J Speech Lang Hear Res* 2012;55:1640–54.
14. Quittner AL, Cruz I, Barker DH et al. Effects of maternal sensitivity and cognitive and linguistic stimulation on cochlear implant users' language development over four years. *J Pediatr* 2013;162:343–8.
15. Hintermair M. Hearing impairment, social networks, and coping: the need for families with hearing-impaired children to relate to other parents and to hearing-impaired adults. *Am Ann Deaf* 2000;145:41–53.
16. Gale E, Berke M, Benedict B et al. Deaf adults in early intervention programs. *Deaf Educ Int* 2021;23:3–24.
17. Yoshinaga-Itano C. Towards a model for the deaf infusion of leadership in early hearing detection and intervention services. The 2015 Libby Harricks Memorial Oration. [Summary available at www.handsandvoices.org/deafhardofhearingchildren/a-new-model-of-deaf-and-hard-of-hearing-infusion, last accessed 20 December 2021]
18. Ching TYC, Dillon H, Leigh G, Cupples L. Learning from the Longitudinal Outcomes of Children with Hearing Impairment (LOCHI) study: summary of 5-year findings and implications. *Int J Audiol* 2018;57(suppl 2):S105–11.
19. Tomblin JB, Harrison M, Ambrose SE et al. Language outcomes in young children with mild to severe hearing loss. *Ear Hear* 2015;36(suppl 1): 76S–91S.

20. Wu C-M, Ko H-C, Tsou Y-T et al. Long-term cochlear implant outcomes in children with GJB2 and SLC26A4 mutations. *PLoS One* 2015;10:e0138575.
21. Moodie SA. Family-centred early intervention: supporting a call to action. ENT and Audiology News, 2018. www.entandaudiologynews.com/features/audiology-features/post/family-centred-early-intervention-supporting-a-call-to-action, last accessed 2 July 2021.
22. Center on the Developing Child at Harvard University. From Best Practices to Breakthrough Impacts: A Science-Based Approach to Building a More Promising Future for Young Children and Families, 2016. https://developingchild.harvard.edu/resources/from-best-practices-to-breakthrough-impacts/, last accessed 2 July 2021.
23. Golinkoff RM, Hoff E, Rowe ML et al. Language matters: denying the existence of the 30-million-word gap has serious consequences. *Child Dev* 2019;90:985–92.
24. Hall ML. The input matters: assessing cumulative language access in deaf and hard of hearing individuals and populations. *Front Psychol* 2020;11:1407.
25. Hirsh-Pasek K, Adamson LB, Bakeman R et al. The contribution of early communication quality to low-income children's language success. *Psychol Sci* 2015;26:1071–83.
26. Huttenlocher J, Waterfall H, Vasilyeva M et al. Sources of variability in children's language growth. *Cogn Psychol* 2010;61:343–65.
27. Moeller MP, Carr G, Seavers L et al. Best practices in family-centered early intervention for children who are deaf or hard of hearing: an international consensus statement. *J Deaf Stud Deaf Educ* 2013;18:429–45.
28. Cawthon SW, Johnson PM, Garberoglio CL, Schoffstall SJ. Role models as facilitators of social capital for deaf individuals: a research synthesis. *Am Ann Deaf* 2016;161:115–27.
29. Hintermair M. Self-esteem and satisfaction with life of deaf and hard-of-hearing people – a resource-oriented approach to identity work. *J Deaf Stud Deaf Educ* 2008;13:278–300.
30. Jackson CW. Family support and resources for parents of children who are deaf or hard of hearing. *Am Ann Deaf* 2011;156:343–62.
31. Watkins S, Pittman P, Walden B. The Deaf Mentor Experimental Project for young children who are deaf and their families. *Am Ann Deaf* 1998;143:29–34.
32. Gale E. Collaborating with deaf adults in early intervention. *Young Exceptional Children* 2021;24:225–36.

Further reading and resources

United Nations. Convention on the Rights of Persons with Disabilities [A/RES/61/106]. www.ohchr.org/en/instruments-mechanisms/instruments/convention-rights-persons-disabilities

United Nations Department of Economic and Social Affairs. Transforming our World: the 2030 Agenda for Sustainable Development. https://sdgs.un.org/2030agenda

Coalition for Global Hearing Health. http://coalitionforglobalhearinghealth.org

Deaf Leadership International Alliance. www.dliaconnect.org

Family-Centered Early Intervention. www.fcei.at

Global Coalition of Parents of Children who are Deaf or Hard of Hearing. www.gpodhh.org

World Federation of the Deaf. https://wfdeaf.org

World Federation of the Deaf. Human rights. https://wfdeaf.org/our-work/human-rights-of-the-deaf/

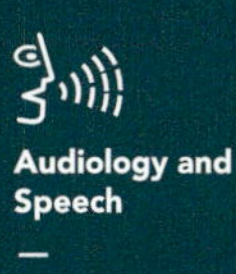

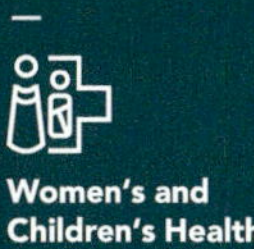

13 Unilateral hearing loss and auditory neuropathy spectrum disorder

Allison L Sedey, Mallene Wiggin, Hsiu-wen Chang and Christine Yoshinaga-Itano

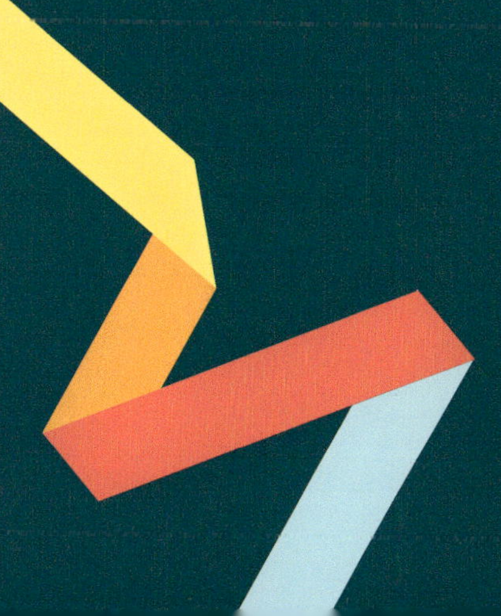

HEALTHCARE

Unilateral hearing loss

UHL is defined as the presence of any type and degree of hearing loss in one ear with normal hearing in the other ear. The potential impact of hearing loss in 'just' one ear is often minimized by both medical professionals and laypersons, with the common misconception that children with UHL will experience little to no listening and/or communication difficulties or delays because they 'have one good ear'. Consequently, this population may receive inadequate medical, audiological and/or educational management.

However, the significant negative impact of UHL is well documented,[1–20] with consequences including deficits and/or delays in speech perception,[1–3] neurological development,[4,5] cognitive function,[6–8] socioemotional skills[9] and language acquisition.[3,10,11] Additionally, children with UHL are at risk for bilateral hearing loss resulting from either recurrent or persistent MEF in the normal-hearing ear and/or the development of PHL in the normal-hearing ear over time.[21–23]

Prevalence. Approximately 1 in 1000 newborns is identified with UHL, with estimates ranging from 0.8 to 2.7 per 1000.[24–27] Differences in prevalence rates may, in part, be attributed to variations in testing protocols, the testing equipment employed and the definition of hearing loss, as well as to regional variations in genetic and environmental risk factors.

Etiologies and risk factors. Although the cause of congenital and early-onset UHL is often unknown, a variety of conditions are associated with it, and additional factors place a child at high risk for UHL (Table 13.1).

Auditory sequelae. The processes involved in hearing with two ears (for example, head shadow effect, spatial release from masking and binaural summation) confer a variety of benefits that are unavailable or diminished for a child with UHL. Thus, this population experiences difficulties with:

- localizing where sound is coming from (which creates significant safety concerns)[1]

- understanding speech in noisy and/or reverberant environments[1–3]
- hearing speech originating on the side of the affected ear[28]
- following conversations that involve multiple people.[28]

For children with UHL, listening is more effortful, and they experience listening fatigue similar to children with bilateral hearing

TABLE 13.1

Common causes of UHL in childhood and additional risk factors

Common causes of UHL

- Structural abnormalities of the outer or middle ear
  - Atresia
  - Ossicular malformations
- Inner ear malformations
  - Cochlear dysplasia
  - Enlarged vestibular aqueduct
  - Auditory nerve absence
  - Auditory nerve deficiencies
- Genetic
  - Associated with a syndrome such as Waardenburg, CHARGE, Stickler
  - Non-syndromic
- cCMV infection
- Meningitis
- Chronic middle ear effusion
- Ototoxic medication

Additional risk factors for UHL

- Admission to the NICU
- Family history of hearing loss
- Craniofacial anomalies
  - Cleft palate
  - Microcephaly
  - Microtia
  - Temporal bone anomaly

loss and significantly greater than for children with normal hearing.[29] Taken together, these wide-ranging listening challenges contribute to significantly poorer speech recognition in both quiet and noisy environments.[1,3]

Neurological sequelae. In addition to difficulties in auditory/speech perception, structural neurological differences – both in the auditory area and other brain structures – have been associated with UHL in both pediatric and adult populations.[4] These differences extend to both cortical growth and synaptic development. Additionally, multiple functional connectivity differences between brain networks involved with cognition, language comprehension and executive function have been identified in children with UHL.[5]

Language and other developmental outcomes. An increasing body of evidence supports the presence of early language delays in many children with UHL[10,11,16–18] that persist through adolescence.[13,14] Scores that fall below age expectations have been noted in a variety of language areas including vocabulary,[10,11,15] morphology and syntax,[15] narrative skills,[20] verbal reasoning[8,14] and language comprehension.[13]

Infancy to preschool. Language challenges in very young children with UHL have been documented, with 41% of a sample population demonstrating delays in preverbal vocalizations[16] and average delays of 5 months noted in producing two-word phrases.[17] In studies of toddlers and preschool-age children with UHL, 25–35% were consistently reported to exhibit significant delays in both receptive and expressive language, even when hearing loss was identified early.[10,11,18] These delays appear to be most pronounced from 24 months of age.[10]

School-age children. Studies of school-age children indicate that, even by adolescence, delays in language persist.[13,14] Similar to the percentage of young children with UHL who demonstrate language delays, 25–40% of school-age children present with academic difficulties as evidenced by being retained a grade in school and/or requiring special education support.[13,14,30–32] A recent study of children from third to tenth grade found that, even after the advent of newborn hearing screening, fewer than 50% of children with UHL scored in the proficient range on a state-wide literacy test. This result was similar to that of children with mild-to-moderate bilateral hearing loss.[19]

Cognitive-linguistic skills and socioemotional wellbeing. In addition to delays in general expressive/receptive language skills and academic development, on average, children with UHL demonstrate significantly lower scores on verbal, full-scale and/or performance intelligence quotient tests.[3,7,8] Reduced accuracy and efficiency in phonological processing and verbal working memory have also been noted.[6] Especially concerning are reports that children with UHL are at risk for social and emotional problems and demonstrate lower quality-of-life scores than hearing peers and peers with bilateral hearing loss.[9]

Factors predictive of language and academic outcomes. Attempts to identify which children with UHL are most likely to exhibit language and/or academic delays have yielded conflicting results. In several studies, children with more significant degrees of hearing loss in the affected ear were more likely to have listening, language and/or educational difficulties.[2,3,11,31] More recent studies have found no association between language outcomes and degree of hearing loss in the affected ear.[10,18] Several older studies found right-ear involvement to be more detrimental to academic achievement than left-ear involvement;[31–33] however, several others more recently reported no ear-specific differences in language measures.[3,10,11,13] Lower levels of maternal education were predictive of poorer language outcomes in one study,[10] but not another.[18] Thus, it is difficult to determine what factors may put a child with UHL at increased risk for language and academic delays.

Treatment/intervention options. Although it is still unclear which intervention practices – in terms of both amplification technology and early intervention practices – are most effective in minimizing the negative sequelae of UHL, intervention in cases of early childhood UHL should include a combination of amplification technology, optimization of the listening environment and FCEI (see Chapter 12). For optimal outcomes, these interventions should be started as early as possible – ideally by or before 6 months of age.[34]

Depending on the type and degree of hearing loss, the following types of hearing technology should be considered:

- conventional hearing aid on the affected ear
- cochlear implant in the affected ear
- contralateral routing of signal amplification system in which a transmitter and microphone is worn on the affected ear and sound is routed to the normal-hearing ear
- bone conduction hearing device
- FM/DM system in which sound is transmitted wirelessly from a speaker's microphone directly to the listener's (typically, normal-hearing) ear.

The listening environment for infants and toddlers with UHL can be optimized by minimizing background noise, reducing the distance from the speaker and directing speech to the affected ear.

FCEI should include encouraging people in the child's environment to use language-enhancing communication strategies such as increasing the quantity and quality of the language input to the child, using communication strategies such as imitation and expansion of the child's utterances and narrating the child's and adult's actions.

Providing optimal care. The first step in creating an effective system of care for children with UHL is acknowledging the significant challenges they face. A multidisciplinary team approach is critical given the wide-ranging issues (medical, hearing, cognitive, language, academic and socioemotional) faced by many children with UHL.[1–20] Prompt medical management of middle ear effusion is important to avoid UHL becoming a temporary, but possibly long-term, bilateral loss. Additionally, physicians can provide information and possibly treatment of outer and middle ear anomalies. As the anchor point of a child's medical care, pediatricians are in an excellent position to make referrals to other members of the care team including audiologists, ophthalmologists (given that vision pathologies commonly co-occur with hearing loss),[35,36] speech pathologists and early interventionists.

Audiological care should include regular hearing tests to monitor transient hearing loss due to middle ear effusion and/or permanent progression of hearing loss in the normal-hearing ear, something that has been reported to occur in 7–17% of children with UHL.[21–23] Early consideration and timely fitting of an amplification device, if appropriate, may minimize some of the negative consequences of UHL.[37–39] Given reports of progressive hearing loss in the affected ear in 21–38% of cases,[21,22] audiological monitoring is critical in determining potentially shifting amplification needs.

Early intervention that is pre-emptive (rather than initiated only after a child demonstrates delays) should begin by 6 months of age to maximize language outcomes.[34] The intervention program should include deafness professionals, parent-to-parent support and involvement of adults whose lived experience includes UHL. For families who opt out of intervention or in areas where children with UHL are not automatically eligible for early intervention services, regular (every 6 months) monitoring of language and other developmental skills using standardized, norm-referenced assessments is critical to identify and address delays in a timely fashion.

Auditory neuropathy spectrum disorder

Auditory neuropathy is a clinical diagnosis used to describe individuals with auditory disorders resulting from dysfunction of the synapse of the inner hair cells and auditory nerve and/or the auditory nerve itself. Children with ANSD can be very different from one another because of the multiple potential sites where lesions can arise. As such, they require specialized procedures for identification and for treatment as habilitation/rehabilitation strategies can be successful but may differ according to the location of the damage to the hearing system.[40] The percentage of the population of children with ANSD that have successful developmental outcomes is as yet unknown.

Prevalence of ANSD ranges from 1–10% of children diagnosed with hearing loss dependent upon the population sampled and the heterogeneity of clinical profiles.[40–45] A higher prevalence of SNHL and ANSD is seen in infants in NICUs,[41–45] and ANSD accounts for up to 30% of SNHL in NICUs. The incidence of ANSD is higher in NICUs than in well-baby clinics.[40,45]

Characteristics of the hearing loss. Bilateral ANSD is found in about 75–79% of affected infants and unilateral ANSD is found in the remaining 21–25%.[45–47] Hearing thresholds can range from thresholds in the normal range to total hearing loss.[44–50] Hearing thresholds frequently fluctuate – there can be over 40 dB variability – and fluctuations are more common in children than in adults.[44–50] Slow deterioration over time at high and mid frequencies has also been reported. Spontaneous improvement may occur when ANSD is associated with anoxia and hyperbilirubinemia in the newborn period.[44–50]

Children with ANSD typically have very poor speech discrimination, even with preserved hearing thresholds, and background noise can further deteriorate residual speech discrimination in children with ANSD.[44–50]

Etiology. The pattern of normal outer hair cell function combined with abnormal neural responses shown by ABR testing places the site of auditory neuropathy to the area of the ear including the inner hair cells, the connections between the inner hair cells and the cochlear branch of the eighth cranial nerve, the eighth cranial nerve itself, and potentially the auditory pathways of the brainstem.[51–53] Neural problems may be axonal or demyelinating and afferent as well as efferent pathways may be involved.

A range of risk factors for ANSD has been identified (Table 13.2).[40]

TABLE 13.2

Risk factors for ANSD

Risk factor	% of cases identified in
Presence of hyperbilirubinemia associated with severe jaundice in the newborn period	50–73%
Prematurity	30–46%
Ototoxic drug exposure	41–80%
Family history of hearing loss	36–38%
Mechanical ventilation	36%
Cerebral palsy	9–15%

Up to 40% of ANSD cases are reported to have a genetic etiology (Table 13.3).[45,54] The problem might also be related to a biochemical abnormality involving neurotransmitter release. The percentages of the population that have specific etiologic causes, whether genetic or environmental factors in utero or after birth, has not been determined.

Structural abnormalities seen in ANSD. Gardner-Barry[55] reported structural abnormalities in 43% of 142 children younger than 10 years seen at the Sydney Cochlear Implant Center in Australia. Of these, 16% had abnormalities on their CT scans, including Mondini deformities, wide internal auditory meatus, dysplastic apical turn, and abnormal vestibule and lateral semicircular canals. Compromised auditory nerves were seen in 20% of the bilateral and 6% of the unilateral ANSD cases.

TABLE 13.3

Genetic causes of ANSD

Non-syndromic

- Non-syndromic autosomal dominant (*AUNA1*, *PCDH9*)
- Non-syndromic autosomal recessive (*OTOF/DFNB9*, Pejvakin [*DFNB59*], *GJB2*)
- X-linked (*AUNX1*)

Syndromic

- Hereditary sensory-motor neuropathy-Lom (autosomal dominant, autosomal recessive, X-linked)
- Leber's hereditary optic neuropathy (mitochondrial)
- Autosomal dominant optic atrophy
- Autosomal recessive optic atrophy
- Mohr–Tranebjaerg syndrome (X-linked recessive)
- Fredreich's ataxia (autosomal recessive)
- Refsum's disease (autosomal recessive)

Teagle[56] reported the preimplant imaging results of 48 children with ANSD and found 23 different abnormalities in 38% of those assessed, the most common of which were:

- periventricular leukomalacia (15%)
- cochlear nerve deficiency in at least one ear (19%)
- Dandy–Walker malformation (4%)
- severe inner ear malformation, including cochlear hypoplasia (6%) and Arnold Chiari type II malformation (2%)
- optoinfundibular dysplasia (2%).

Diagnosis. Most newborn hearing screening programs use both OAE and aABR to test a baby's hearing. If infants are screened with OAE technology first, or if programs use only OAE screening, children with ANSD will pass the hearing screen and remain unidentified.[40]

To ensure identification of infants with ANSD, aABR screening should always be used in NICUs. Screening with aABR should also be carried out in well-baby clinics.

Children with ANSD are characterized by:

- an absent or abnormal middle ear muscle reflex
- present OAEs
- absent or abnormal ABR thresholds
- presence of a polarity-reversing cochlear microphonic followed by typically absent or significantly aberrant wave forms.

Middle ear muscle reflex tests how well the ear responds to loud sounds. In a healthy ear, loud sounds trigger a reflex and cause the muscles in the middle ear to contract. Infants with ANSD require much louder sounds to trigger a reflex.

Otoacoustic emissions testing measures how well the outer hair cells in the cochlea function. With ANSD, the OAE response is normal.

Auditory brainstem response testing measures whether the auditory nerve transmits sound from the inner ear to the lower part of the brain and how loud sounds have to be for the brain to detect them. With ANSD, there is an absent or abnormal response. Diagnostic ABR should include a search for a cochlear microphonic.

If an ANSD diagnosis is made, additional tests are required, including:[40]

- otologic evaluation with imaging of the cochlea and auditory nerve (CT and MRI) to see if the auditory nerve is present in both ears and if there are any inner ear abnormalities
- genetic testing to determine cause and, if necessary, provide appropriate treatments
- neurological testing by a neurologist to assess peripheral and cranial nerve function
- ongoing communication assessment to monitor speech and language development, evaluate the effectiveness of treatment and modify it when appropriate
- ophthalmology assessment to determine if there is any associated vision loss.

Auditory neuropathy and comorbidities. Due to the high incidence of ANSD in the NICU, ANSD may coexist or be associated with a multitude of other disorders that may impact communication development, including cognitive, neurological and perceptual disorders, speech-motor disabilities or visual disabilities. Socioemotional disorders, such as autism, are also seen.

The prevalence of these comorbidities in children with ANSD has not been well studied but Uhler et al.[46] reported that 57% of children with ANSD had hearing loss with additional disabilities. Significant cognitive delays were about twice to three times more common in children with bilateral ANSD than in children with bilateral SNHL.

Treatment/intervention options. The therapeutic interventions that are most effective for children with ANSD with specific characteristics are not yet clear, but some general therapeutic approaches include:[40,46,49]

- providing signal-to-noise maximization with FM listening devices
- amplification via hearing aids and cochlear implants
- speech/language intervention, which may include both auditory and visual communication strategies (for example, cued speech, sign language).

Key points – unilateral hearing loss and auditory nerve spectrum disorder

- UHL affects approximately 1 in 1000 newborns and has a significant negative impact on speech perception, neurological development, cognitive function, socioemotional skills and language acquisition.
- There is conflicting evidence on which factors predict delays in language and academic development in children with UHL.
- Early intervention, ideally by or before 6 months of age, is important for optimal outcomes in children with UHL.
- ANSD is a result of damage to the inner row of hair cells in the ear, or to the synapses between the hair cells and the auditory nerve, or damage to the auditory nerve itself.
- Infants with ANSD can be missed if only OAE testing is used for screening.
- ANSD can be associated with multiple comorbidities, including cognitive, neurological and perceptual disorders, speech-motor disabilities, visual disabilities and socioemotional disorders.

References

1. Reeder RM, Cadieux J, Firszt JB. Quantification of speech-in-noise and sound localisation abilities in children with unilateral hearing loss and comparison to normal hearing peers. *Audiol Neurootol* 2015;20(suppl 1):31–7.
2. Ruscetta MN, Arjmand EM, Pratt SR. Speech recognition abilities in noise for children with severe-to-profound unilateral hearing impairment. *Int J Pediatr Otorhinolaryngol* 2005;69:771–9.
3. Lieu JE, Karzon RK, Ead B, Tye-Murray N. Do audiologic characteristics predict outcomes in children with unilateral hearing loss? *Otol Neurotol* 2013;34:1703–10.
4. Heggdal POL, Brännström J, Aarstad HJ et al. Functional-structural reorganisation of the neuronal network for auditory perception in subjects with unilateral hearing loss: review of neuroimaging studies. *Hear Res* 2016;332:73–9.

5. Jung ME, Colletta M, Coalson R et al. Differences in interregional brain connectivity in children with unilateral hearing loss. *Laryngoscope* 2017;127:2636–45.
6. Ead B, Hale S, DeAlwis D, Lieu JEC. Pilot study of cognition in children with unilateral hearing loss. *Int J Pediatr Otorhinolaryngol* 2013;77: 1856–60.
7. Purcell PL, Shinn JR, Davis GE, Sie KC. Children with unilateral hearing loss may have lower intelligence quotient scores: a meta-analysis. *Laryngoscope* 2016;126:746–54.
8. Martínez-Cruz CF, Poblano A, Conde-Reyes MP. Cognitive performance of school children with unilateral sensorineural hearing loss. *Arch Med Res* 2009;40:374–9.
9. Borton SA, Mauze E, Lieu JEC. Quality of life in children with unilateral hearing loss: a pilot study. *Am J Audiol* 2010; 19:61–72.
10. Sedey AL, Yoshinaga-Itano C, Clark A, Wiggin M. Language outcomes of children with unilateral hearing loss: a multi-state perspective. Early Hearing Detection and Intervention Conference 2015, Louisville, KY, USA, 2015: oral presentation.
11. Sedey A, Stredler-Brown A, Carpenter K. Language outcomes in young children with unilateral hearing loss. National Workshop on Mild and Unilateral Hearing Loss 2005, Breckenridge, CO, USA, 2005:28.
12. Anne S, Lieu JEC, Cohen MS. Speech and language consequences of unilateral hearing loss: a systematic review. *Otolaryngol Head Neck Surg* 2017;157:572–9.
13. Lieu JE, Tye-Murray N, Karzon RK, Piccirillo JF. Unilateral hearing loss is associated with worse speech-language scores in children. *Pediatrics* 2010;125:e1348–55.
14. Fischer C, Lieu J. Unilateral hearing loss is associated with a negative effect on language scores in adolescents. *Int J Pediatr Otorhinolaryngol* 2014;78:1611–17.
15. Sangen A, Royackers L, Desloovere C et al. Single-sided deafness affects language and auditory development – a case-control study. *Clin Otolaryngol* 2017;42:979–87.
16. Kishon-Rabin L, Kuint J, Hildesheimer M, Ari-Even Roth D. Delay in auditory behaviour and preverbal vocalization in infants with unilateral hearing loss. *Dev Med Child Neurol* 2015;57:1129–36.
17. Kiese-Himmel C. Unilateral sensorineural hearing impairment in childhood: analysis of 31 consecutive cases. *Int J Audiol* 2002;41:57–63.

18. Fitzpatrick EM, Gaboury I, Durieux-Smith A et al. Auditory and language outcomes in children with unilateral hearing loss. *Hear Res* 2019;372:42–51.
19. Yoshinaga-Itano C, Mason C, Wiggin M et al. Reading proficiency trends following newborn hearing screening implementation. *Pediatrics* 2021;148:e2020048702.
20. Young GA, James DG, Brown K et al. The narrative skills of primary school children with a unilateral hearing impairment. *Clin Linguist Phon* 1997;11: 115–38.
21. Fitzpatrick EM, Al-Essa RS, Whittingham J, Fitzpatrick J. Characteristics of children with unilateral hearing loss. *Int J Audiol* 2017;56:819–28.
22. Uwiera TC, DeAlarcon A, Meinzen-Derr J et al. Hearing loss progression and contralateral involvement in children with unilateral sensorineural hearing loss. *Ann Otol Rhinol Laryngol* 2009;118:781–5.
23. Lin PH, Hsu CJ, Lin YH et al. Etiologic and audiologic characteristics of patients with pediatric-onset unilateral and asymmetric sensorineural hearing loss. *JAMA Otolaryngol Head Neck Surg* 2017;143:912–19.
24. Berninger E, Westling B. Outcome of a universal newborn hearing-screening programme based on multiple transient-evoked otoacoustic emissions and clinical brainstem response audiometry. *Acta Otolaryngol* 2011;131:728–39.
25. Bussé AML, Hoeve HLJ, Nasserinejad K et al. Prevalence of permanent neonatal hearing impairment: systematic review and Bayesian meta-analysis. *Int J Audiol* 2020;59:475–85.
26. Ghirri P, Liumbruno A, Lunardi S et al. Universal neonatal audiological screening: experience of the University Hospital of Pisa. *Ital J Pediatr* 2011;37:16.
27. Iwasaki S, Hayashi Y, Seki A et al. A model of two-stage newborn hearing screening with automated auditory brainstem response. *Int J Pediatr Otorhinolaryngol* 2003; 67:1099–104.
28. Priwin C, Jönsson R, Magnusson L et al. Audiological evaluation and self-assessed hearing problems in subjects with single-sided congenital external ear malformations and associated conductive hearing loss. *Int J Audiol* 2007;46:162–71.
29. Bess FH, Davis H, Camarata S, Hornsby BWY. Listening-related fatigue in children with unilateral hearing loss. *Lang Speech Hear Serv Sch* 2020;51:84–97.
30. Lieu JE, Tye-Murray N, Fu Q. Longitudinal study of children with unilateral hearing loss. *Laryngoscope* 2012;122:2088–95.
31. Bess FH, Tharpe AM. Case history data on unilaterally hearing-impaired children. *Ear Hear* 1986;7:14–19.

32. Oyler RF, Oyler AL, Matkin ND. Unilateral hearing loss: demographics and educational impact. *Lang Speech Hear Serv Sch* 1988;19:201–10.
33. Jensen JH, Johansen PA, Børre S. Unilateral sensorineural hearing loss in children and auditory performance with respect to right/left ear differences. *Br J Audiol* 1989;23:207–13.
34. Yoshinaga-Itano C, Sedey AL, Wiggin M, Chung W. Early hearing detection and vocabulary of children with hearing loss. *Pediatrics* 2017;140:e20162964.
35. Gruber M, Brown C, Mahadevan M, Neeff M. Hearing loss and ophthalmic pathology in children diagnosed before and after the implementation of a universal hearing screening program. *Isr Med Assoc J* 2019;21:607–11.
36. Batson S, Kelly K, Morrison D, Virgin F. Ophthalmologic abnormalities in children with congenital sensorineural hearing loss. *J Binocul Vis Ocul Motil* 2019;69:126–30.
37. Purcell PL, Jones-Goodrich R, Wisneski M et al. Hearing devices for children with unilateral hearing loss: patient- and parent-reported perspectives. *Int J Pediatr Otorhinolaryngol* 2016;90:43–8.
38. Briggs L, Davidson L, Lieu JEC. Outcomes of conventional amplification for pediatric unilateral hearing loss. *Ann Otol Rhinol Laryngol* 2011;120:448–54.
39. Hassepass F, Aschendorff A, Wesarg T et al. Unilateral deafness in children: audiologic and subjective assessment of hearing ability after cochlear implantation. *Otol Neurotol* 2013;34:53–60.
40. Hayes D, Sininger Y. Guidelines for Identification and Management of Infants and Young Children with Auditory Neuropathy Spectrum Disorder. Guidelines Development Conference at NHS 2008, Como, Italy, 2008.
41. Boudewyns A, Declau F, van den Ende J et al. Auditory neuropathy spectrum disorder (ANSD) in referrals from neonatal hearing screening at a well-baby clinic. *Eur J Pediatr* 2016;175:993–1000.
42. Uus K, Bamford J. Effectiveness of population-based newborn hearing screening in England: ages of interventions for identified babies and profile of cases. *Pediatrics* 2006;117: e887–93.
43. Berg AL, Spitzer JB, Towers HM et al. Newborn hearing screening in the NICU: profile of failed auditory brainstem response/passed otoacoustic emission. *Pediatrics* 2005;116:933–8.
44. Rance G. Auditory neuropathy/ dys-synchrony and its perceptual consequences. *Trends Amplif* 2005;9:1–43.
45. De Siati RD, Rosenzweig F, Gersdorff G et al. Auditory neuropathy spectrum disorders: from diagnosis to treatment: literature review and case reports. *J Clin Med* 2020;9:1074.

46. Uhler K, Heringer A, Thompson N, Yoshinaga-Itano C. A tutorial on auditory neuropathy/dyssynchrony for the speech-language pathologist and audiologist. *Semin Speech Lang* 2012;33: 354–66.
47. Meleca JB, Stillitano G, Lee MY et al. Outcomes of audiometric testing in children with auditory neuropathy spectrum disorder. *Int J Pediatr Otorhinolaryngol* 2020;129:109757.
48. Chandan HS, Prabhu P. Audiological changes over time in adolescents and young adults with auditory neuropathy spectrum disorder. *Eur Arc Otorhinolaryngol* 2015;272:1801–7.
49. Rance G, Beer DE, Cone-Wesson B et al. Clinical findings for a group of infants and young children with auditory neuropathy. *Ear Hear* 1999;20:238–52.
50. Vignesh SS, Jaya V, Muraleedharan A. Prevalence and audiological characteristics of auditory neuropathy spectrum disorder in pediatric population: a retrospective study. *Indian J Otolaryngol Head Neck Surg* 2016;68:196–20.
51. Kraus N, Bradlow AR, Cheatham MA et al. Consequences of neural asynchrony: a case of auditory neuropathy. *J Assoc Res Otolaryngol* 2000;1:33–45.
52. Berlin CI, Bordelon J, St John P et al. Reversing click polarity may uncover auditory neuropathy in infants. *Ear Hear* 19:37–47.
53. Dowley AC, Whitehouse WP, Mason SM et al. Auditory neuropathy: unexpectedly common in a screened newborn population. *Dev Med Child Neurol* 2009;51:642–6.
54. Manchaiah VKC, Zhao F, Danesh AA, Duprey R. The genetic basis of auditory neuropathy spectrum disorder (ANSD). *Int J Pediatr Otorhinolaryngol* 2011;75:151–8.
55. Gardner-Barry K. Cochlear implants in infants and children with ANSD: experiences at the Sydney Cochlear Implant Center. Diagnosis and Management of Auditory Neuropathy Spectrum Disorder Conference 2012, St Petersburg, FL, USA, presented paper, 2012.
56. Teagle HFB, Roush PA, Woodard JS. Cochlear implantation in children with auditory neuropathy spectrum disorder. *Ear Hear* 2010;31: 325–35.

Further reading and resources

Unilateral hearing loss

American Speech Language Hearing Association. Unilateral hearing loss in children. www.asha.org/public/hearing/unilateral-hearing-loss-in-children/

Boys Town National Research Hospital. What is unilateral hearing loss? www.boystownhospital.org/knowledge-center/unilateral-hearing-loss

Hands & Voices. Unilateral hearing loss tips for parents. www.handsandvoices.org/articles/early_intervention/uni_loss_tips.html

Tharpe AM. Unilateral hearing loss in children: current perspectives. www.hearingreview.com/hearing-products/hearing-aids/speech-noise/unilateral-hearing-loss-in-children-current-perspectives

Auditory nerve spectrum disorder

BabyHearing.org. Auditory neuropathy spectrum disorder. www.babyhearing.org/auditory-neuropathy-spectrum-disorder

Hearing Loss Association of America. Auditory neuropathy. www.hearingloss.org/hearing-help/hearing-loss-basics/auditory-neuropathy/

Hood LJ. Auditory neuropathy: what is it and what can we do about it? LSU Health Sciences Center; https://web.archive.org/web/20060709015953/http:/www.medschool.lsuhsc.edu/Otorhinolaryngology/deafness_article1.asp

Interacoustics. Cochlear microphonics CM, 2016. www.interacoustics.com/guides/test/abr-tests/cochlear-microphonics-cm

Morlet T. Auditory neuropathy spectrum disorder and (central) auditory processing disorder. *Deaf-Blind Perspectives* 2010;17:1–5.

National Institute on Deafness and Other Communication Disorders. Auditory neuropathy. www.nidcd.nih.gov/health/auditory-neuropathy

Index